Health Care in
France and Germany

Health Care in France and Germany: Lessons for the UK

David G. Green
Benedict Irvine

Civitas: Institute for the Study of Civil Society
London

First published December 2001
Civitas
The Mezzanine, Elizabeth House
39 York Road, London SE1 7NQ
email: books@civitas.org.uk

ISBN 1-903 386-17-9

Typeset by Civitas
in New Century Schoolbook

Printed in Great Britain by
Hartington Fine Arts Ltd
Lancing, West Sussex

Contents

Authors

David G. Green is the Director of Civitas. His books include *Power and Party in an English City*, Allen & Unwin, 1980; *Mutual Aid or Welfare State?*, Allen & Unwin, 1984 (with L. Cromwell); *Working-Class Patients and the Medical Establishment*, Temple Smith/ Gower, 1985; *The New Right: The Counter Revolution in Political, Economic and Social Thought*, Wheatsheaf, 1987; *Reinventing Civil Society*, IEA, 1993; *Community Without Politics*, IEA, 1996; *Benefit Dependency*, IEA, 1998; *An End to Welfare Rights*, IEA, 1999; *Delay, Denial and Dilution*, IEA, 1999 (with L. Casper); and *Stakeholder Health Insurance*, Civitas, 2000.

He wrote the chapter on 'The Neo-Liberal Perspective' in *The Student's Companion to Social Policy*, Blackwell, 1998.

Benedict Irvine is Project Manager of the Civitas Health Unit. After studying law he completed a master's degree in comparative European public administration at the Catholic University of Leuven, Belgium. Before joining Civitas he worked as a researcher in the European Parliament. His areas of interest include citizen participation in public policy making, particularly in health care and social housing provision. He also holds degrees in music.

Acknowledgements

A special thank-you must go to all our interviewees—in Paris, Munich, Berlin and London—who willingly gave up so much of their time. For the assistance given at the beginning of this project, we thank the social affairs staff at the French and German Embassies in London. We are also grateful to Dr Reinhard Busse of the European Observatory on Healthcare Systems and Professor Juergen Wasem of the University of Greifswald, who provided very welcome technical advice about German health care. Finally, we must thank those who participated in the anonymous refereeing process, whose constructive comments have certainly improved the finished product. Naturally, all remaining errors are our own.

Introduction

'I saw a long queue, so hopped on the tube and went to a different practice.'
'She was rather ill-tempered so I never went back.'
'The facilities were drab, so I went to a different one next to my office.'
'I felt rushed at his practice so didn't go back.'

These were some of the remarks made by German consumers of healthcare in surveys conducted for this publication. If anything, the French were even more demanding. One French woman we spoke to told us that she had found some of the nursing staff in a French public hospital 'rude and uncaring'. We pressed for the details and discovered that her main objection was that the nurses had not knocked before entering her private room. Such high expectations were typical in both France and Germany. In the UK our expectations are much lower.

There are many publications which compare healthcare systems and analyse the differences between them, but the special focus of this study is on health care in France and Germany from the vantage point of the individual consumer. What are the realities of each system for ordinary people trying to earn a living and raise a family? And what are the lessons for Britain?

Chapter 1 describes what our French and German interviewees told us. Separate chapters are then devoted to the systems in France and Germany, and in the concluding chapter, we suggest some lessons for public policy in Britain.

We have not tried to describe every aspect of the French and German systems in the manner of a textbook. Rather we have focused on elements of each system from which we think the NHS may have the most to learn. We have been guided by the following main questions.

First, do individuals have any control over how much of their own money is spent on health care? How visible is their contribution? As we shall see, there are significant differences between systems. In France there is a mixture of user charges and social insurance. Germany's system is also based on social insurance, but with far fewer fees at the time of use. In both countries social insurance payments are highly visible on pay slips, but in Britain we have no way of calculating how much of our taxes goes to the NHS.

Second, which organisation receives the money taken from individuals and whose interests are served by this third-party payer? In Britain the Treasury takes the taxes and treats the money as its own. How do France and Germany differ?

Third, does the system encourage doctors to serve their patients? In Britain paternalism is the rule, though mitigated by a professionalism which often encourages doctors to put their patients first. Are France and Germany any different?

Fourth, who owns the hospitals and other healthcare institutions? What incentives do the owners or managers have to serve customers?

Finally, what standard of care is available for the poorest members of society, including the unemployed? Is it clearly an inferior standard? Or is it a standard also enjoyed by middle-income earners?

1

France and Germany:
The Consumer's View

We begin with the evidence from international surveys of patient satisfaction. Based on the regular Eurobarometer survey, Dr Mossialos of the London School of Economics has reported public attitudes throughout the 15 EU member states (see Table 1, p. 4).[1] One question asked was: 'In general, would you say you are very satisfied, fairly satisfied, neither satisfied nor dissatisfied, fairly dissatisfied or very dissatisfied with the way health care runs in [country]?'

There is a difference of 26 percentage points between the UK and France: 41 per cent of Britons were very or fairly dissatisfied, only 15 per cent of the French, and only 11 per cent of Germans.

The 1996 Eurobarometer survey also asked respondents the following question: 'Now, I will read you four statements about the way health care runs in [country]. Which one comes closest to your own point of view?'

- On the whole, health care in [country] runs quite well.

- There are some good things and minor changes would make it work better.

- There are some good things but only fundamental changes would make it better.

- Health care in [country] runs so badly that we need to rebuild it completely.

Table 2 (p. 5) shows that while 56 per cent of those in the UK sought fundamental change or a complete rebuild of their healthcare system, only 19 per cent of Germans sought such reform—a difference of 37 percentage points. Again, there is a huge disparity between France and the UK: 26 percentage points. Nearly 30 per cent of the French wanted fundamental changes or a complete rebuild, compared with 56 per cent of Britons. Moreover, the view of the French was well founded. In comparison with other European countries, France performs well by almost all standard population and health status measurements.[2] For example, when the World Health Organisation controversially ranked the world's healthcare systems in 2000, France came top of the league.[3]

Such were the quantitative results of national opinion surveys. Are they consistent with the opinions of French and German consumers when questioned more closely about their personal experiences?

Table 1
Public Satisfaction with Healthcare Systems, 1996 (%)

Country	Very and fairly satisfied	Neither satisfied nor dissatisfied	Very and fairly dissatisfied	Other
Austria	63.3	27.6	4.7	4.5
Belgium	70.1	19.9	8.3	1.6
Denmark	90.0	3.8	5.7	0.5
Finland	86.4	7.0	6.0	0.6
France	65.1	18.7	14.6	1.6
Germany	66.0	21.4	10.9	1.7
Greece	18.4	27.0	53.9	0.6
Ireland	49.9	17.4	29.1	3.6
Italy	16.3	23.1	59.4	1.3
Luxembourg	71.1	16.1	8.9	3.9
Netherlands	72.8	8.8	17.4	1.0
Portugal	19.9	19.2	59.3	1.5
Spain	35.6	34.0	28.6	1.8
Sweden	67.3	16.7	14.2	1.9
UK	48.1	10.0	40.9	1.0

Source: Mossialos, 1997.

Table 2:
Public Viewpoint on Healthcare Reforms, 1996 (%)

Country	Runs quite well	Minor changes needed	Fundamental changes needed	Rebuild it completely	Other
Austria	40.2	33.5	18.0	3.3	5.0
Belgium	41.7	34.0	16.5	2.9	4.9
Denmark	54.4	37.2	5.7	1.8	1.0
Finland	38.9	51.6	7.7	0.6	1.2
France	25.6	40.9	24.6	5.0	3.9
Germany	36.9	38.5	16.7	2.2	5.7
Greece	3.8	25.5	44.2	25.0	1.6
Ireland	19.4	30.7	25.6	16.9	7.4
Italy	3.4	15.1	43.8	33.1	4.5
Luxembourg	31.9	43.9	13.3	2.5	8.4
Netherlands	31.0	46.0	17.6	3.5	1.9
Portugal	3.6	19.4	38.3	31.8	6.9
Spain	14.1	30.4	34.0	13.5	7.9
Sweden	28.5	44.1	21.8	3.4	2.2
UK	14.6	27.4	42.0	14.0	2.0

Source: Mossialos, 1997

French Consumers

We begin with some first-hand accounts of the French system based on interviews with French citizens conducted in December 2000.[4] Chapter 2 then looks at the system and explains how it empowers patients, despite the French predilection for dirigisme.

Secretary

When we spoke to her Madame Rouge was a secretary who lived in Paris. She was married with two children. Now in her early forties, she and her husband both worked. They earned above the *Couverture Maladie Universelle* (CMU) threshold and therefore did not qualify for free cover. Both of their employers pay contributions into the national insurance fund which covers about 80 per cent of the population: *Caisse Nationale d'Assurance Maladie des Travailleurs Salariés* (CNAMTS)—health insurance organisation for salaried workers.[5] To supplement their medical cover—largely because their children were often sick—they also paid into a *mutuelle*.[6] The package they chose was a comprehensive one covering almost all medical costs not reimbursed by national insurance. Until recently, they had attended a local family doctor (*médecin de famille*) to ensure continuity of care for their children. When the children had reached their teens, the family tended to choose a variety of sometimes more expensive *conventionné* generalists and specialists (see p. 41 for details).

Mme Rouge told us about three of her recent experiences of the French system.

Abscess on Tonsil

Suffering from throat pain, Mme Rouge went to a local pharmacy to buy some throat pastilles. In France these are classified as 'comfort' drugs and do not qualify for reimbursement. The next day, the pain had worsened and soon she couldn't swallow. She knew an ear, nose and throat specialist, as her daughter had visited him on many occasions when she was younger, and asked for an appointment as quickly as possible. The following day, in the course of a thorough 25-minute examination, the specialist found an abscess on a tonsil. The specialist lanced the abscess immediately and gave Mme Rouge a prescription for antibiotics which she obtained at a pharmacy around the corner. She did not have to return to the specialist for any further treatment but said she would go to him again because he solved the problem so quickly.

As a sector 1 *conventionné* specialist (see below p. 42) the consultation fee was FF 150 (about £15) and the antibiotics cost FF 30 (about £3).[7] Seventy per cent of the consultation fee was reimbursed by the sickness fund and the remainder by her *mutuelle*. Having attached the white sticker (given to her by the pharmacist) to her prescription form, she was also fully reimbursed for the antibiotics—65 per cent by the sickness fund and 35 per cent by the *mutuelle*.

Gynaecological Problem

Mme Rouge was referred to a specialist by her preferred sector 1 private GP, who recommended a 'world-renowned specialist' whom he knew. Unusually, she had to wait a week for an appointment because the specialist was at a conference in the Far East. This short wait was not a concern for her, because she thought she was in the hands of the best in the world.

At her initial consultation Mme Rouge had an x-ray, a biopsy, and a full explanation of exactly what the specialist recommended and was going to do. She felt that she was given ample high-quality information. Moreover, she was offered a choice over whether to go ahead with certain elements of her treatment and felt that the decision-making process had been a real partnership.

On making an appointment, the hospital she had chosen to attend sent a fact sheet to Mme Rouge which included the name of the operation, the day and time of surgery, the pre-operative requirements, a check list of what might happen as a result of the operation (including side-effects), a list of what would happen in the event of side-effects, and an emergency contact number in case any of the above ill-effects were serious.

She had a private room in the hospital and said that the care she received was excellent.[8] The expenses for her treatment and hospital stay were covered fully by the sickness fund and the *mutuelle*, though having chosen to be treated in a private '*clinique*' she had to pay rather more for her treatment before claiming her refund.

In the past Mme Rouge had lived for a period with her husband in London, and had required gynaecological treatment while there. Mme Rouge was shocked at the difference in attitudes towards patients—the very curt treatment and interpersonal relations that she experienced as an NHS patient left her feeling patronised and unaware of exactly what was happening to her and why.

Skiing Accident

While skiing in the Alps, Mme Rouge tore a ligament in her leg. She went to see a local GP without an appointment—presenting her social security number to show that she was entitled to care.

The GP said that an x-ray was required, and recommended a local specialist (10km away). Mme Rouge attended the specialist's surgery that afternoon and as a result was given a letter to give to a surgeon on her return to Paris, explaining what was required. The (*sector 2*) specialist's fee was FF 380 (about £38.00)—of which 70 per cent of FF 150 was reimbursed.[9] The majority of the balance was then reimbursed by the *mutuelle*. The *conventionné* generalist's fee was FF 110 (about £11), 70 per cent of which was reimbursed by the sickness fund, and the remainder by her *mutuelle*.

After a successful operation in a Parisian public hospital, she was prescribed 20 hour-long sessions of physiotherapy —at FF 75 each, the total payable at the end of the course, was FF 1,500 (about £150). However, before going ahead with this treatment she had to request authorisation to be reimbursed from the local *Caisses Primaires d'Assurance Maladie* (CPAM)—this abbreviation is a bit of a mouth-full in French, so it is more affectionately known as the '*sécu*') of the CNAMTS. Reimbursement was duly granted and the CPAM paid 70 per cent and her *mutuelle* the rest.

Mme Rouge was very satisfied with the health-care system in France, and her only complaint was the length of time it took for her sickness fund to reimburse expenses.[10]

Teacher

We interviewed Mme Bleu who was aged 31 and lived in Paris. She was single with no dependants and worked full-time as a school-teacher, earning more than the CMU threshold and paying into the general national sickness fund for teachers—*Mutuelle Générale de l'Éducation Nationale* (MGEN). Like Mme Rouge, she had supplementary insurance to cover co-payments *(ticket modérateur),* in her case one specifically targeted at civil servants. She was short-sighted and so chose a relatively expensive package that gave good coverage for spectacles. Mme Bleu attended a *médecin de famille* when she was young and living with her parents in Burgundy.[11] Now, having left home and as a fairly mobile person, she preferred to shop around and changed doctors regularly—relying on advice from friends and colleagues. Mme Bleu expected that she would return to a *médecin de famille* if she had children. She also had some indirect experience of the new *référent* system (see pp. 42-43) through her elderly parents who had used one in rural Burgundy. Unlike many of her friends, who thought it a complete failure, she thought the *référent* system was good for elderly patients who perhaps didn't have the necessary 'word-of-mouth' contacts to make an informed choice of doctor, nor perhaps the ability or the desire to actively 'shop around'.

Mme Bleu told us about some of her recent health-related experiences in France.

Mixed Experiences—Shortage of Nurses and Paramedics?

On suffering anaphylactic shock, Mme Bleu's retired mother (in a coma) was admitted to a 'resuscitation centre'. However, before admission there was a problem with the emergency transport. In France the public can choose to call the *Service d'Aide Médicale Urgente* (SAMU) (highly skilled paramedics) or the *pompiers-médicaux* (emergency first aid). Not realising the seriousness of her mother's condition, Mme Bleu called the *pompiers* who took 30 minutes to arrive (it being a fairly rural area) and then recognising the gravity of situation decided that they shouldn't do anything and so called the SAMU. After another 30 minutes the SAMU arrived and were excellent, but that didn't stop the family worrying about the delay in her treatment.

Once admitted, the public resuscitation service was excellent in all respects—well staffed and highly effective. However, on leaving 'resuscitation' the conditions in (a different) public hospital during recuperation were less satisfactory. There appeared to be a shortage of nursing staff—which may explain why she said that nurses were sometimes rude and appeared uncaring. For example, she had a private room and objected to the nurses' habit of entering without knocking.

So why did the family pick that hospital? Her mother was given the option of going to another hospital two hours away that may have been more suitable, but the family was adamant that easy access to their mother was of greatest importance. Despite these concerns, the food was good—patients were offered four courses from a menu that changed regularly.

Following her release from hospital, Mme Bleu's mother followed courses of physiotherapy at her local hospital. Unfortunately, her appointments were cancelled regularly and sometimes without explanation—further evidence of a local shortage of specialists. Because she is retired, the expenses for her mother's treatment were covered by the CNAMTS.

Asthma

As an asthmatic (a condition classified nationally as a 'chronic and long-term condition') Mme Bleu is entitled to what is often called 'cent pour-cent'—100 per cent cover for all illness related to her asthma.[12] She explained that once diagnosed with the condition, patients are given a form proving their entitlement to free cover. When further consultations or repeat prescriptions are required the patient simply takes the form and avoids the need for advance payment.

Contraception

Mme Bleu's personal experiences of obtaining the contraceptive pill in France and the UK (where she had studied for a while) are also revealing. In France, new recipients of the pill have their blood cholesterol monitored for the first three months. Surprised and concerned that such testing did not happen in the UK, she concluded that French doctors are rather more concerned with the health of their patients.[13]

Back pain

Mme Bleu developed back pain while working for a period in London a few years ago. After waiting nearly two weeks to see a GP, she was referred for a scan but was told she could not have an appointment under the NHS for three months. She had a forthcoming meeting in Paris and so decided to use that opportunity to have a scan. Only two weeks before the meeting, Mme Bleu called the Hôpital St Antoine and arranged for the scan to be carried out on the day and at exactly the time she wanted it. Once processed, the results were sent immediately to her old *médecin de famille* in Burgundy, who telephoned her in London to say that no action was required. All of this happened around four weeks before the date of the appointment she had been offered in London.

Despite her concerns, Mme Bleu was largely content with the French system of health care. She was also quite certain that, if she lived in the UK again, she would have any necessary treatment performed in France, not the UK.

Civil Servant

Our third interviewee, Madame Vert, was in her mid-fifties and worked in Paris as a civil servant. She was married with two children at university. She earned above the CMU threshold and therefore did not qualify for free care. She was a member of the national social security scheme for civil servants. She also paid for a top-level *mutuelle* package as she was a regular hospital user (eight operations so far), who expected privacy. Designed for civil servants, this *mutuelle* package cost 2.5 per cent of her salary—roughly £50 per month. By combining the National Health Insurance (NHI) reimbursement with that of the *mutuelle*, nearly 100 per cent of all hospital costs (even in private clinics) were covered. When her children were younger she went to a *médecin de famille* regularly. Now, she tended to choose a variety of *conventionné* generalists and specialists, normally going to those recommended by friends and family for specific problems.

Mme Vert told us about the following experiences.

Pharmacies

Found on virtually every street corner, Mme Vert told us that she regarded pharmacies as the primary source of basic information about health care in general and about the healthcare system. The high quality information provided free of charge had been particularly useful when her children were younger.

Counselling / Psychology

These services are used extensively by the French. In her case she attended a clinic for some time after her marriage broke up. Mme Vert said that, throughout France, counselling sessions must always be paid for in cash—with reimbursement claimed later. She thought this fact might dissuade the less well-off (perhaps those who needed it most) from seeking such care.

Surgery

Mme Vert used to live and work as a French civil servant in London. Having had good experience of GPs in Britain she was told that she needed a serious operation. This was duly planned, the appropriate tests were done and an appointment fixed for surgery. As instructed, the day before she was due to be admitted, Mme Vert telephoned the ward and was told, to her dismay, that her operation had been cancelled because there was no bed available.

This caused Mme Vert considerable concern because she had given notice to her employer that she would be absent, and a replacement for her had already been found. She went back to work, spoke to her French boss who suggested that she go to France for the operation—after all, she had full national insurance medical cover and a *mutuelle* to cover the costs not paid by her social security medical insurance.

Mme Vert then telephoned her *médecin de famille* in Paris and explained what had happened. He suggested a specialist whom she telephoned from London to explain the story so far—what tests she had had and what operation she needed. The following day (Sunday) Mme Vert flew to Paris, where she attended the private clinic on Monday for tests. (These were required to avoid serious mistakes and to protect against legal action for error. A French specialist must be able to justify all operations on strictly medical grounds.) The operation was carried out on the Tuesday morning. She then rested at the clinic for a week, and was able to return to work in London as previously planned.

She said that she had received this type of high quality, quick treatment in each of her seven other operations. The costs of each had been fully covered by the state sickness fund and her *mutuelle*.

Unnecessary Investigation

On a more negative side, she had had an experience of what she regarded as needless investigation in France. A few years ago, she was certain that her son had an infection and went to a (*non-conventionné* - see p. 41) GP simply seeking a prescription. However, the doctor insisted on numerous tests and then decided that her son had a virus. On receipt of a bill for around £70, she refused to pay—a decision that the GP apparently accepted. She was most unhappy with the behaviour of the GP, and it is difficult confidently to explain his behaviour. It is possible that he was being careful about the prescriptions he handed out, or he may have been making as much money as he could out of a patient whom he knew to be fully covered by a *mutuelle*. Mme Vert thought the latter explanation more likely and never went back to that doctor.

German Consumers

Secretary

Our first German interviewee was Frau Grun, aged 45 and an administration assistant in Munich. She was married with two school-aged children, one of whom was disabled. Frau Grun was part of the mandatory health insurance system—at the moment she is a member of the *Techniker*

Krankenkasse.[14] She paid about DM 150 (about £60) per month and her employer paid DM 150—which covers almost everything except prescriptions. When asked, she did not know exactly what percentage of her salary it was, but said it was clearly marked on her pay-slips. Frau Grun said that she was satisfied with the service her family received and, if she had the choice, certainly would not opt for supplementary private insurance, or private care. She has no reason to want to go private, because she thought public facilities were the best, and, in any case, with a family it would be too expensive to opt for private cover.

When Frau Grun was younger she was in the general local fund—the *Allgemeine Ortskrankenkasse* (AOK).[15] Then she moved to the USA with her husband and children for a period (and had great difficulty obtaining care for their disabled child). On their return to Germany she looked after the children at home and her husband, a scientist, had to rejoin his old insurer, the *Techniker*. The whole family was covered by his policy. Then Frau Grun started work again as a clerical worker. At the time she was obliged to join the *Deutsche Angestellten Krankenkasse* (DAK) insurance fund for salaried employees.[16] She felt the DAK was satisfactory, but, as soon as membership of *Krankenkassen* was liberalised in 1996, she changed to the *Techniker* because it was cheaper and had better extra benefits.[17]

Although there are quite a few small *Techniker* insurance offices around the city of Munich, Frau Grun was rarely in contact with the insurer, but had been recently to obtain prior agreement before certain dental work for her children. She explained that recently the *Krankenkassen* had cut back on the use of dental braces—if payment is to be made by the insurer, braces may only be used in cases of medical need and not for cosmetic purposes. In the dental field, and certain others where co-payments must be made for medical checkups, there is a financial encouragement to have regular checkups. For example, if attendance has been regular, 90 per cent of cost will be paid by the insurer, whereas if attendance has been less regular, only 80 per cent will be paid. Frau Grun responded to such incentives.

Competition and Choice

Germans change doctors frequently and Frau Grun certainly regarded herself as a consumer of healthcare services. She mentioned that before finding her current GP she had been to one who had made her feel rushed and slightly unwelcome.[18] She never went back. She had also changed gynaecologist because she had not liked the manner of the first one.

However, she had not changed doctors regularly, because she valued the personal relationship gained from attending one doctor, and thought the health care received might be better—more holistic. Her current GP was the nearest, and always seemed caring and very down-to-earth, with a relaxed and chatty atmosphere in the consulting room. She liked him immediately and so did not need to shop around nor to ask friends or colleagues. She thought that this type of service was common, because doctors aim to provide a service that will attract the highest paying private clients, and that level of service trickles down to all patients. She would not return to a doctor who was paternalistic.

Frau Grun thought that German patients were more empowered, and took greater responsibility for their own care, than in other countries. As a result, Frau Grun said she took self-diagnosis pretty seriously.

On the whole she would go to a GP (the same one repeatedly) before attending a specialist—with her *Uberweisung* (referral form) but she would go directly to see a gynaecologist, or an eye specialist. If she was not sure what was wrong with her, but did not think her GP could help, she would go to an *Internist*—a general adult internal specialist. If one of her children fell ill they would go straight to the *Kinderspezialist*.[19]

Her GP and her regular network of specialists each keep their own medical records. When asked whether, as a consequence of this division of medical records, there was a risk of conflicting treatments from different specialists, she thought there was such a risk, but in her experience physicians were careful to check what (if any) other medical treatments were being carried out.

Frau Grun would seek second opinions if she had any doubt about a diagnosis, or if she wanted to be doubly sure before submitting to treatment. In one case, she saw three different specialists before deciding to go ahead with an operation.

A GP Visit

Typically she might wait about ten minutes before seeing the doctor for an appointment that lasted around 15 minutes. She described her latest visit to her GP. Suffering back pain when she arrived at work one morning, she rang her usual GP, and arranged an appointment for two hours later. When she arrived, there was nobody else in the surgery—she showed her *Chip-karte* (credit-card sized smart card—proving entitlement to statutory health insurance to the receptionist, who would put it in the machine. By manipulation of her back and questioning, the doctor tried to isolate the source of the problem. The GP explained that if the problem did not recede by the time of her next appointment (the following week) she would need an x-ray, and might also need an injection—so the doctor tested for potential allergic reaction. Frau Grun was prescribed some tablets for her discomfort, and when she left the surgery a computer-generated prescription form was waiting for her at the reception. She took this form to the independent pharmacist across the road, and obtained her drugs. She returned to work just before lunchtime.

At the next appointment, as the pain had cleared up, there was no need to have an x-ray, but had there been, the GP had the facilities in his surgery. Throughout this procedure Frau Grun paid only DM 9 (about £3) for the pain killing prescription.[20] On submitting an invoice (quarterly) according to the standard scale of fees, the doctor would be paid (via the regional association of physicians) by the insurer.

A Hospital Visit

On a separate occasion, in the course of an appointment, her private gynaecologist diagnosed a problem that required hospital-based testing and treatment. The specialist telephoned a local hospital and was given a list of possible dates for admission within the coming month.

Frau Grun had to send a form to her insurance company, *Techniker*, agreeing to pay for treatment. The insurance company had no preference for one hospital or another and Frau Grun chose where to go. On arrival at the hospital she presented her insurer's authorisation for treatment and was shown to her public ward with four beds.

Inside the hospital, Frau Grun thought the standards of treatment and equipment were excellent. Hospital cleanliness was also very good. Having lived abroad for a while, she thought the hospitals in Germany were of the same very high standard as those in the US. Her only criticism was that hospital food was not the best. In the course of her treatment, she only paid for the daily 'hotel expenses' charge (DM 17—about £6). The GKV insurance company paid for her treatment. Having treated Frau Grun, the hospital-based specialist would be paid by the insurer in accordance with an official scale.

Accident and Emergency

Frau Grun told us briefly about her son's recent visit to A&E. Having fallen and cut his hands, Frau Grun and her husband drove to the local hospital where her son was seen immediately in casualty. There was no waiting. Her husband had to show evidence of their insurance, but that did not get in the way of treatment. Her son's hand was cleaned and stitched, and, as their GKV insurance cover included dependent children and emergency hospital treatment, the Grun's paid nothing.

Teacher

When interviewed, Frau Schwartz was married, aged 55 with two children, neither of whom was dependent. As a school teacher, she was *Beamte* (permanent civil servant), and *de facto* obliged to take out private health cover.[21] Many different companies offer private health insurance, and Frau Schwartz chose her current insurer—*BBV*

Krankenversicherungs, based on the price. Her husband, also a teacher, was covered under a separate private policy with the same insurer. In cases where both parents are working teachers, Frau Schwartz explained that children would be covered by the policy of one of the parents. However, private insurance contribution rates are lower for *Beamten* than those paid by salaried workers earning above the income threshold.

As a rule Frau Schwartz contacts the insurer for reimbursement purposes only. If a medical bill is for less than DM 1,000 she would pay it in full.[22] She then sends the bill to BBV, which reimburses her very quickly. Indeed, if reimbursement were slow they would consider changing insurer.

Frau Schwartz's family used two different types of GP: single practice and group practice. Her solo practitioner was a migraine expert who had an assistant and four rooms including a small laboratory. She explained that group practices typically had two or more resident doctors, with many rooms with more modern and better equipment than the average single practice. Her whole family has had a long-term relationship with the single practitioner, which she values. But she would sometimes choose to go to the better-equipped larger practice (recommended to her by a work colleague).

Frau Schwartz found both of her GPs by word of mouth. In choosing a GP, she took into account the quality of care and the reputation of the physician as perceived by herself and her friends or colleagues, then qualities such as friendliness and accessibility. Because of her children, she particularly valued GPs who would do home visits at any time of the night.

Illustrating the nature of her relationship with doctors, Frau Schwartz told us that the solo GP sent patients birthday cards, hailed the Schwartzs as friends in the street, and always asked about the family in consultations: he could not be less paternalistic. Also (partially by way of drumming-up business she suggested) he invited patients to lectures on certain topics—the most recent was on osteopathy. These events would take place in a bar, and patients would listen to a presentation and then have a discussion. However, Frau Schwartz did not think this was a common phenomenon.

Because she was satisfied with the service, she had not changed GP regularly. However, she had frequently changed her dentist, and some years earlier she had obtained three specialist opinions before having a small back operation.

Frau Schwartz had built up a relationship with a couple of good local doctors and, on the whole, she said she would go to a GP before a specialist. If however, she had a skin condition she would go directly to a *Dermatologist*, with an eye problem to an *Augenarzt* (specialist eye doctor) and for anything to do with ears, nose or throat she would visit a specialist. For a mammogram she would go directly to a gynaecologist, and, when they were younger, if one of her children became ill they would attend specialist *Kinder-arzten*. As a rule she would go to the same set of specialists, but felt less of a tie to them, and so would be more likely to change if not entirely satisfied.

A Typical Private Practice Visit

Frau Schwartz usually telephoned in advance to make an appointment. On arrival she would tell the receptionist that she was privately insured, show her credit-card sized membership card and give her name and address. In the course of a typical visit the doctor would spend some time asking about her health generally, the family, work, and so on. During examination Frau Schwartz always asked for and was given ample information about tests, diagnoses and options for treatment. With a possible wait of ten minutes, a normal visit might last 30 minutes in total. She would leave with a referral note and/or a prescription—for which she had to pay a small amount and then claim reimbursement from her insurer. Some time after the appointment an invoice would be sent to her home. She would pay it, then send the invoice to her insurer for a refund.

A Typical Hospital Visit

Frau Schwartz chose to be treated as a private patient (with access to the head of department and private accommodation) in a large public hospital. She thought this would result in the best quality of care in pleasant surroundings.

In her experience, the head of the hospital department came round the hospital daily to see his private patients. Examinations would be carried out by less experienced doctors first, and their diagnosis would then be checked by the professor, who would subsequently fully examine the patient himself. She thought that the professor saw patients for what were pretty trivial matters, but even if the professor was very busy, a private patient—having paid for insurance and who pays medical bills directly—would expect to see him. Frau Schwartz did say that she had been asked on one occasion whether she would mind being examined by a less experienced medic. She did not mind, but thought this would be a rare occurrence because Germans typically want the best, and expect to get it if they have paid for it.

For certain lengthy or expensive procedures, prior approval of the private insurer must be sought. For example, Frau Schwartz had to obtain approval before going into hospital for allergy testing, which required 15 days as an in-patient. The prices were approved and the insurer agreed to pay for treatment in a two-bed room. Frau Schwartz did not go into detail about this allergy testing. She explained that before a private patient leaves hospital in Germany they are given a very specific long bill by the finance department—every injection, plaster, and so on is included. Subject to the amount owing, an invoice would be sent to either the patient or the insurer. As her allergy testing was an expensive procedure, the hospital (physician) sent the bill directly to her insurance company for payment.

Frau Schwartz thought German health care was expensive, but that generally people she knew were happy to pay because care was very good and there was no waiting or rationing.[23] The right to choose and change both doctors and hospitals means that most doctors try to provide the best service possible. As a school teacher with a similar professional standing, she thought that most people she knew counted doctors among their friends, and so would expect to receive high quality service without waiting.

Student

We interviewed Herr Weiss who was unmarried and from Hannover. Students who are financially dependent on their parents are usually covered by the same policy as their parents. While at university, Herr Weiss was privately insured under his father's *Debeka* insurance. (He had private insurance because his father earned above the GKV income threshold and chose to buy private insurance.) He explained that both the private and statutory insurers offer students cheap cover (students might expect to pay DM 95-105 per month— about £30) for those who choose not to be covered by their parents' policy.

Herr Weiss rarely visited a doctor, but would decide whether to go to a GP or a specialist depending on his symptoms—the *Sportarzt* (sports medicine specialist) after a skiing fall, an *Augenarzt* for eye problems, and a GP or *Internist* for most other things. In choosing a specialist, he would rely on recommendations from friends or family (when back at home). If he liked the quality and style of treatment delivery, he would probably go back to the same practice, gradually building up a group of his chosen physicians. Suspecting their motive for treatment to be financial, he had changed dentist on quite a few occasions.

Experience of Private Practice Visits

On the recommendation of a course colleague, Herr Weiss attended a well-equipped group practice where GPs do ECGs, immunisations, take blood and have the facilities to carry out tests in their own small laboratory. Administration is computerised, and the GP sends any referrals by fax directly to specialists—often those working in the same building.

On feeling ill, he would usually telephone and ask: 'Can I come now'. The answer had always been 'yes'. Waiting times were very short: even without an appointment he has never waited for longer than 40 minutes. As a private patient, Herr Weiss thought he generally benefited from fast track treatment. This opinion may or may not be valid in his case. He thought this was a negative feature of the 'dual system' and competition between doctors. However, he noted that not all doctors gave priority to private patients.[24]

Following treatment, private patients are invoiced by the physician. As a student, the system is the same. His parents receive an invoice, pay, and then send a copy of the invoice to the insurer, which reimburses them. However, if the treatment were expensive (on one occasion he had had a bill for over DM 1,000 for back treatment) the insurer would pay the provider directly.

Pensioner

All wage- and salary-earners are subject to compulsory pension insurance which comprises invalidity insurance, old-age insurance, and survivor's insurance.[25] Statutory health insurance is also compulsory for German pensioners, who remain with the fund they were contracted with at the time of their retirement. As people get older, they tend to change insurer with less frequency: this is particularly the case for the privately insured, as premiums for elderly new members are higher.

There is the same entitlement to benefits in kind for the pensioner and for his or her dependants. Pensioners contribute according to the general contribution rate of the sickness fund, with half paid by the pensioner (six per cent) and half by the statutory pension fund (six per cent).[26] Thus, the pension fund takes over that portion of health insurance cover previously paid by the employer.[27]

Treatment By a Private Practice Specialist

The following series of events relates to the elderly English mother (Mrs Englischer) of an interviewee, Mr Englischer. Mrs Englischer was treated under the E111 scheme, which entitles UK citizens to the same treatment as any German would receive. The E111 scheme is affiliated to the AOK insurer.

During a short visit in summer 2000, Mr Englischer's mother slipped, fell to the pavement and injured herself. The village where he lived in the foothills of the Alps has many orthopaedic or sports medicine specialists. Because she was in pain, he made an appointment for the same day without attending a GP first, because it seemed obvious that his mother would be referred to a specialist.

At the reception they handed in their E111 form proving entitlement to insurance cover from AOK. They then went straight in to see the specialist who, after discussing what had happened, arranged an x-ray. The specialist came back in 15 minutes with the result, explained what damage the fall had done, and asked more about her medical history. Mrs Englischer was prescribed painkillers, advised to have some physiotherapy when she returned home, and for support and protection, was prescribed a corset. Using his laptop, the specialist sent a request to his regular supplier and organised an appointment for fitting the following morning. The specialist also recommended a further check-up before her return to the UK.

They left the office, picking up the prescription at reception, and went to the nearby pharmacy to collect the painkillers—which cost DM 11 (about £3.50).

The following morning, Mr Englischer and his mother had the corset fitted and the fitter asked them to return the following day between 10 a.m. and 12 noon, if the corset was uncomfortable. The corset was 'cutting' a bit, so the Englischers called in at about 11 a.m. and the fitter adjusted the corset accordingly.

Three days later she returned to the specialist for a check-up. She had another x-ray and was offered a prescription for more painkillers. The specialist insisted that she must see her GP when she returned home to the UK. The only charges were for the painkilling drugs.

Unemployed Person Who Has Never Worked

We interviewed Herr Grau who had spent some time studying in the UK. When he returned to Germany he was unemployed. Because he had never worked, he was unable to join one of the GKV insurers, so received *Sozialhilfe* (benefit from the social welfare office) and *Sozialamt* healthcare cover.[28] The local *Sozialamt* had an agreement with the local AOK fund so he received health cover 'in association with AOK' but not directly from AOK. Ultimately, the *Sozialamt* paid for his health care. To access care Herr Grau received a special *Krankenschein* (a certificate proving entitlement for treatment) from the local AOK.

In practice Herr Grau thought that choice was restricted for the German poor. Most obviously, there was no choice of insurer, nor *de facto* choice between the use of public and private hospital facilities. However, unemployed patients have the same freedom of access to private practice specialists as other GKV and PKV insured, and they make their choice of GP and specialist in the same way, relying on recommendations from friends and family, weighing up the pros and cons of accessibility, typical length of appointment and so on. Less positively, Herr Grau reported that, while there was little if any stigma involved in having your sickness fund contributions paid by the *Sozialamt* insurance, his choice of doctor was effectively restricted because he had a *Krankenschein*, and not a *Chip-karte*. Some doctors would not take patients with the *Krankenschein* because they considered the paperwork to be too much of a burden.

In similar vein, unlike those with *Chip-karten*, *Sozialamt* patients with a *Krankenschein* must hand them to a physician for a whole financial quarter. Thus, it was not possible to go to more than one GP or specialist of the same specialty in the same three-month period. In particular, this restricted the seeking of second opinions, although the choice was only restricted to the extent experienced by all Germans prior to the issuing of *Chip-karten* in 1996.

Finally, although the quality of care received by the unemployed should be the same, *Sozialamt* patients have to obtain prior authorisation for many more procedures than their statutorily insured neighbours. Thus, speedy access to treatment is less freely available to those on *Sozialhilfe*.

To receive health care, Herr Grau typically made an appointment, or simply went to the physician (usually a GP) of his choice, gave his special AOK *Krankenschein* to the receptionist and received treatment, just like anyone else. Unless unemployment was the result of invalidity, Herr Grau thought a doctor would not necessarily know that a patient was unemployed. He thought that stigma/discrimination was an issue for some unemployed seeking access to healthcare services, but that this was attached to being a *Sozialamt* benefit recipient or AOK subscriber ('by association'), rather than to unemployment *per se*. For example, he said that normally patients would wait five to ten minutes before seeing the doctor, but occasionally they might wait up to an hour, particularly if insured by AOK or on *Sozialhilfe*. He suggested this was perhaps because doctors in certain practices had less, or even no interest in treating AOK patients. He thought that privately insured patients were more likely to take priority for some physicians, but this would not be a general rule—particularly in poorer areas with a larger proportion of patients in receipt of *Sozialhilfe*.

Following treatment, at the end of the financial quarter, Herr Grau said his doctor would send his invoice to the *Sozialamt*. While unemployed, and in receipt of welfare benefits, Herr Grau did not pay for prescriptions.

Freelance/Self Employed

Finally, we spoke to 28-year-old Herr Braun, a British national, engaged to and living with a German in former East Berlin. As a self-employed language teacher, his salary varied each month. He cannot join a GKV fund, because he had never been employed in Germany. The same rule applies to university graduates who start their own businesses immediately on completion of their studies. Herr Braun chose to purchase an AOK private plan for *Freiwillegen*—those professionals and the self-employed who can either choose to 'go private' or are not able to be GKV members. He had shopped around and found that the AOK plan was the only one he could afford.

Herr Braun paid 15.9 per cent of his gross income and could not deduct the cost as a business expense. Unlike the employed who pay half, he had to pay all of his health insurance contribution, as well as pension and the other mandatory insurances. Along with many other self-employed people in Germany he found the social protection contributions punitive and a real disincentive to work harder.

His former GP in the old East Berlin (a single-handed practice with no receptionist) used to complain that it was not worth his while to treat AOK private patients and urged him to change insurers. Herr Braun considered this and investigated the possibilities, using the list of insurers that the doctor had given to him, but again found other private insurers' contribution rates to be punitively high—DM 500 (about £170) per month for example, as opposed to AOK's DM 210 (about £70).[29]

Herr Braun contacts his insurer infrequently—only when seeking prior approval for procedures that are not explicitly covered by his policy. In such cases, AOK replies specifying what percentage reimbursement will be paid following treatment.

In choosing a GP doctor or specialist, Herr Braun relied on recommendations. Unless he was absolutely certain of the source of a medical problem, on the whole he would go to a GP before going to a specialist. His reason for this was partly financial and partly to guarantee medically holistic treatment. As a paying patient, he thought it would be cheaper in the long run to risk one appropriate referral from a GP, than a string of referrals from private specialists.

Herr Braun had not changed doctors regularly, but had recently changed, partially owing to the pressure his former East German doctor put on him and partially because the facilities and décor were better in his new multiple-physician practice. He did not seek second opinions as to do so would be expensive (he pays the bills before reimbursement) and he has found a GP he trusts.

Herr Braun described a recent private practice visit to us. Suffering back pain, he made an appointment for the following day at a new group practice near his workplace. On arrival, he showed proof of insurance and gave his address to the medical receptionist. He waited for a few minutes and then saw the GP who quickly recognised the nature of the problem, prescribed a painkiller and advised that he should see an orthopaedic specialist. The GP generated a referral form, faxed it directly to a 'recommended' specialist based in the same building and then made a number of appointments in the following weeks for Herr Braun to see the specialist. Herr Braun said his medical records were e-mailed to the specialist. He paid the pharmacist DM 13 (about £4.50) for his prescription and received an invoice in the post for his GP appointment. He paid this in full and then forwarded the invoice to AOK, which reimbursed 100 per cent of the cost.

Herr Braun had not used in-patient hospital services, so had not really exploited the potential for private treatment cover. Again, owing to the expense of treatment, he said he would be unlikely to pay for upgrades to the most expensive accommodation—feeling that treatment on the public wards would be sufficient. He told us about a recent A&E visit.

Experiencing what he thought were serious chest pains at 2 a.m. one Saturday night, and urged to act by his fiancée, he phoned a taxi and went to the local A&E. On arrival, he went to reception and showed his insurance identification. He was seen very quickly—only waiting for about ten minutes. The doctor gave him an ECG, and while showing Herr Braun the results explained that there was nothing serious wrong with him, suggesting perhaps he was experiencing a trapped nerve or intercostal pain. The doctor prescribed a series of six, half-hour long massages at an external private physiotherapist—at a cost of DM 13 (about £4.50 per session). This had to be paid in cash, as, he explained, physiotherapists do not send invoices. He was in and out of the hospital A&E in just over half an hour. He had complete confidence in the diagnosis and, despite the brusqueness of the doctor, was impressed by the standard of care received.

No money changed hands during the A&E visit. Herr Braun received a detailed bill later which he sent to the insurer for reimbursement. His insurance policy also paid for travel to hospital a certain number of times per year.[30]

2

France: The System

Political and Administrative Structures

Following the Algerian crisis, the Fifth Republic, a unitary presidential democracy, was established by a referendum in 1958. In unitary systems sovereignty lies exclusively with the central government. Sub-national authorities, whether regional or local, may make and implement policy but they do so by permission of the centre.

France has a multi-party system, but possesses a very strong executive figure—the president.[1] The parliament consists of two chambers: the National Assembly and the Senate. The former, with 577 directly elected deputies who represent their constituencies for five years, is politically more important than the Senate of 321 members, who are elected by representatives of local organisations and serve for nine years.[2]

Despite central *dirigisme*, since the 1980s France has established a system of co-ordinated, decentralised and regional government. In 1986 the 22 regions acquired competencies in economic, social and cultural development, tourism and regional infrastructure. There is also an elected socio-economic council in each region which acts as an advisory council and includes representatives of employers, employees, farmers and social organisations—the 'social partners'. French localities (96 *départments*), while possessing considerable autonomy in practice, form part of a uniform system of administration applying across the country. The municipalities are administered by an elected council, voted in every six years. This council selects the mayor, who has executive responsibility for public health at a local level.[3]

Social Insurance

Regulation—With a Heavy Touch

France has a reputation for state direction and protectionism, but the French healthcare system is based on a compromise between two conflicting ideologies, egalitarianism and liberalism. All citizens are said to be equal; yet, choice and competition are fiercely protected. Consequently, the French system is a unique blend of private and public. It is mainly financed by social insurance but there is also a significant supplementary insurance sector.[4] About two-thirds of hospital beds are in the public sector with the remainder split between the for-profit and non-profit private sectors.

Along with much of the developed world, the French authorities have been trying to control government spending on health care. Slowing economic growth, rising unemployment and continued population ageing have contributed to rising health expenditure and resultant deficits in statutory health insurance.[5] Successive French governments have, with differing degrees of resolve, tried to implement a variety of cost-containment policies aimed at limiting supply, restricting coverage and suppressing demand. While these efforts have been met by much public discontent and typically militant opposition by most of the medical unions, budget equilibrium for the general scheme was reached in 1999.[6]

Everyone who is employed in France is subject to French social security legislation and liable to pay contributions to the French schemes for pensions, sickness (including health care) and unemployment.[7] The national social security scheme is divided into four 'branches' for those employed in industry or trade: sickness 'and maternity benefit, insurance in the event of death, and invalidity insurance; accidents at work and occupational diseases; old-age; and family. We are concerned with the first branch only, under which the employed, unemployed and pensioners as well as their dependants are entitled to medical treatment.

The right to medical assistance for the poor was established in 1893, followed soon after by legislation to support and encourage social insurance provision by mutual societies. Health insurance was made compulsory for all employees in 1930, and extended to farmers in 1961 and the self-employed in 1966. The French model of social insurance looks complicated. One commentator has remarked that the multiplicity of payers and the variety of providers, each with a degree of independence from government, 'leaves their public/private status unclear'.[8]

The national health insurance (NHI) system guarantees universal access to health care for the whole population. The system is administered in schemes according to occupation. About 80 per cent are covered by the general scheme *Caisse Nationale d'Assurance Maladie des Travailleurs Salariés* (CNAMTS). These are mainly salaried workers belonging to the commercial and industrial sectors and their families.[9] The CNAMTS covers the country through a system of 16 regional and 133 local funds, each of which is a self-governing unit, with a management board composed of an equal number of representatives of employers and trade unions.[10] Seventeen other basic funds cover specific occupational groups: agricultural workers, independent professions, civil servants, medical doctors and students.[11]

Employers are required to complete the necessary formalities to ensure social security coverage. Once completed, a registration card is issued with an insurance number, a *carte vitale* (see p. 37). This number is required every time an individual applies for benefits. In order to qualify for cover, a person must have either worked for a certain number of hours in the month before treatment, or have paid contributions above a certain threshold based on the minimum wage.

The French government has the prime responsibility for the health and social protection of all its citizens and regulates the healthcare system closely. Specifically, the state underwrites the training of health personnel; defines working conditions; regulates the quality of health service organisations; monitors safety; regulates the volume of health services supply; and oversees social protection. It manages and intervenes in the methods of financing: setting tariffs, determining coverage of the population, and regulating relations with health service producers.[12]

Since the 1996 Juppé reforms, the *parliament* has had ultimate responsibility for setting the objectives and the annual budget for the social security scheme. The *High Committee of Public Health*, chaired by the Health Minister, defines health objectives in an annual report. The *National Health Conference*, composed of a cross-section of health agencies, proposes the priorities. Finally, there are the *Conférences Régionales de Santé,* which analyse local health needs and establish the priorities for public health.[13]

Authority over the regulation of finance and coverage rests with the powerful Ministry of Finance, as well as the Ministry of Social Affairs and Employment.[14]

In addition, there are 22 regional health and social affairs bureaux (DRASS), whose main tasks are to plan health and social services within annual budget controls, to monitor the 'health plans' which establish the number of hospital beds by specialty and area, to establish rules for the installation of costly medical equipment, and to control inpatient treatment facilities and the regional sickness funds.[15]

The CNAMTS is responsible for the general development of sickness insurance while the regional funds co-ordinate capital development. French residents register at the local CPAM—affectionately known as the *'sécu'* of the CNAMTS. The *'sécu'* are responsible for the reimbursement of claims, benefits, sanitary and social care in their area, and various preventive measures. The CPAM offices we visited in Paris were similar to our local social security offices in this country: grey, unattractive, crowded, dirty.

The *Caisses Régionale d'Assurance Maladie (CRAM)* assume responsibility for the CPAMs in their area. They manage the prevention of workplace accidents, occupational illnesses, and the administration of social and sanitary programmes.[16] In addition, new regional organisations have been established—*Unions Régionales des Caisses d'Assurances Maladie* (URCAM)—to co-ordinate social insurance administration at a regional level.[17]

Finance

In 1999 total healthcare expenditure was among the highest in Europe at 9.4 per cent GDP. This was divided between NHI (75.5 per cent), supplementary private insurers (12.1 per cent—the greater part being provided by mutual societies), general taxation (about 1.1 per cent), while the remainder (11.3 per cent) was paid by patients.[18]

The national insurance scheme was financed through employer and employee payroll contributions. Contribution levels for the national insurance *caisses* are fixed by the government.[19] The insurers are non-government, non-profit agencies, which owe their allegiance to employers and employees. Premiums are charged as a percentage of income and the total cost is nearly 20 per cent of payroll, including the employer's and employee's contribution.

Recently the regime has reduced reliance on payroll contributions. Employers still pay 12.8 per cent of an employee's salary to the health insurer, but the contribution rate for employees has been lowered from 5.5 per cent at the end of 1997 to 0.75 per cent in 2001. Simultaneously, an earmarked social security tax, (*Contribution Sociale Généralisée* [CSG]) on employment and capital income has been introduced. By broadening the base of social security contributions the government aims to take financial pressure off employers. The appropriate contributions are deducted by the employer and subsequently paid alongside the employer's contribution to *Union de Récouvrement des cotisations de Sécurité Sociale et d'Allocations Familiales* (URSSAF), and immediately distributed to relevant social security 'branches'. These deductions are clearly marked on French employee pay-slips. (An example of a French pay-slip may be found on the next page.)[20]

Example of Part of a French Pay-slip

LIBELLE	BASE	EMPLOYEUR Taux	EMPLOYEUR Montant	SALARIE Taux	SALARIE Montant	S/TOTAL
SALAIRE DE BASE	151,67			90,59	13740,00	13740,00
CONGES PAYES du 02/06/00 au 02/06/00	-/20			687,00	-687,00	
INDEMNITES DE CONGES PAYES					-687,00	
SUBSTITUTION					1990,00	
BRUT	144,09					15730,00
BRUT SOUMIS						15730,00
CHOMAGE TRA (ASSEDIC)	15730,00	3,970	624,48	2,210	347,63	
ASF TRA (ASSEDIC)	15730,00	1,160	182,47	0,800	125,84	
RDS-CSG NON DEDUCTIBLE (URSSAF)	14943,50			2,900	433,36	
CSG DEDUITE (URSSAF)	14943,50			5,100	762,12	
MALADIE REGIME GENERAL (URSSAF)	15730,00	12,800	2013,44	0,750	117,98	
VEUVAGE (URSSAF)	15730,00			0,100	15,73	
ASSURANCE VIEILLESSE (URSSAF)	15730,00	8,200	1289,86	6,550	1030,32	
VIEILLESSE 2 (URSSAF)	15730,00	1,600	251,68			
ALLOCATIONS FAMILIALES (URSSAF)	15730,00	5,400	849,42			
FONDS D'AIDE AU LOGEMENT (URSSAF)	15730,00	0,100	15,73			
FONDS D'AIDE LOGEMENT >9 SALARI (URSSAF)	15730,00	0,400	62,92			
ACCIDENT DU TRAVAIL (URSSAF)	15730,00	1,520	239,10			
FONDS NATIONAL DE GARANTIE (ASSEDIC)	15730,00	0,200	31,46			
RETRAITE COMPLEMENTAIRE TRA.2 (UPS)	15730,00	5,250	825,83	3,500	550,55	
TAXE SUR TRANSPORTS (URSSAF)	15730,00	2,500	393,25			
PARTICIPATION A LA CONSTRUCTION (OCIL)	15730,00	0,450	70,79			
FORMATION (FONGECIF)	15730,00	1,200	188,76			
TAXE 3 SUR LES SALAIRES (FISC)	8773,33	9,350	820,31			
TAXE 2 SUR LES SALAIRES (FISC)	3475,00	4,250	147,69			
TAXE 1 SUR LES SALAIRES (FISC)	15730,00	4,250	668,53			
TOTAL RETENUES			8675,72		3383,53	-3383,53
CARTE ORANGE	265,00			0,50	132,50	132,50
TICKET REST.	20,00			-19,00	-380,00	-380,00
				NET A PAYER		12098,97

Message   Net a Payer en Euro (1 Euro = 6,55957 FF) : 1844,48

The Expanding Role of Supplementary Health Insurance

Supplementary insurance typically pays for healthcare costs that are not covered by NHI. Insurance schemes are offered by scores of organisations around the country. There are three types of provider: provident societies, *mutuelles*, and private commercial insurers. Some of these are tailored to certain professions, while others are general national insurers. People either take out individual personal plans (of which there is a very wide range available), or join an employer-based scheme (usually negotiated at a favourable rate) if one is available.

Table 3
Supplementary Health Insurance as a Percentage
of All Health Care Finance. 1975-1995

Percentages covered by supplementary insurance	1975	1995
Expenditure for medical goods and services	3.8	6.8
Hospital Care	1.1	2.1
Total ambulatory care*	6.2	10.8
Services provided by office-based doctors	7.4	10.5
Dental Services	5.2	13.6
Pharmaceuticals	6.4	12.4

* Some policies also cover hospital charges—such as the *forfait journalier*—the daily hotel expenses charge.

Source: Mossialos, *Health Care and Cost Containment in the EU*, 1999.

The increasing role of *assurance complémentaire* has enabled the French people to avoid healthcare rationing, which the French find culturally unacceptable. Among others, Redwood in *Why Ration Health Care?* observes that the public has shown a clear preference for paying supplementary insurance premiums rather than unrecoverable fees at the point of use.[21] In 2001 about 87 per cent of the population paid for supplementary insurance—rising from 31 per cent in 1960.[22]

Direct Payment by Patients

The concept of *médecine libérale* dates from the late 1920s. It assumes that payment *(avance de frais)* is made directly by the patient to the doctor at the point of use according to the services provided. It is seen as protecting the patient's freedom to choose a doctor, and the doctor's freedom of prescription or practice.[23] These three principles—personal payment, choice of doctor and freedom of practice—remain fundamental to the French healthcare system.

The sense of responsibility created by direct payment is regarded as important, even though a proportion of the payment is reimbursed, and despite the fact that the majority of people pay for additional insurance to cover any co-payments. Supporting the view that co-payment acts as a brake on consumption, many of those French people we spoke to are conscious that 'free' care may encourage wasteful and frivolous use of health services.[24] They typically disapprove because 'the many' end up paying for 'the few'.

The sums reimbursed to patients are calculated as a percentage of the tariffs which are set annually, resulting in the *'ticket modérateur'*. The co-payments detailed in MISSOC and the government information service *'vosdroits'* are:

- Consultation fees during hospitalisation: 20 per cent.

- Hospital treatment: 20 per cent in most cases.

- Doctors' fees (specialists and general practitioners): 30 per cent.

- Paramedic's fees and charges for laboratory tests: 35 per cent.

- Medicines with a blue 'vignette' (see p. 47): 65 per cent.

- Medicines with a white 'vignette' (see p. 47): 35 per cent.

- For irreplaceable (vital) or costly drugs: 0 per cent.

- For non-prescribed ease/comfort drugs: 100 per cent.

- Other expenses, including transport costs: 30 per cent.

- There is also a daily hospital charge (*forfait hospitalier*) of FF 70 (about £7).[25]

However, if the patient requests it, there are a number of occasions when the regime makes a direct payment to the provider, comprising the amount that would have been reimbursed (*tiers-payant*—the literal translation of which is 'one-third to pay'). Therefore the patient only pays the *ticket modérateur*. This applies to much payment for pharmaceuticals and public hospital care, and unsurprisingly tends to be taken advantage of more often by those on lower incomes.[26]

Private hospitals are not bound by the same official rates and the patient is usually expected to pay fees before reimbursement. This obviously affects the accessibility of the less well-off to health care offered by these providers. Whatever type of hospital patients attend, there is a fixed charge per day (*taut/forfait journalier*), to cover accommodation, food etc. Certain categories of people are exempt from this flat-rate charge including children, those receiving maternity benefit, and war pensioners.

For certain services, including much dentistry, prostheses and long courses of physiotherapy, advance approval from the appropriate fund must be granted. This is obtained through the local CPAM office.

In certain circumstances, patients qualify for payment exemption—100 per cent *prise en charge* ('taken care of')—by the NHI.[27] Also called '*cent pour-cent*' (100 per cent), it means that the relevant sickness fund pays the full cost. There are three broad reasons for such exemption from co-payment:

- *Medical Condition*. To protect people from exposure to very high expenditure owing to serious illness or expensive treatments. The list of conditions covered includes: cancer, diabetes and AIDS. A diabetic with flu, for example, will be fully reimbursed for prescriptions relating to diabetes, but will be subject to the same rules as other citizens for the treatment of flu.

- *Nature of services provided/treatments required.* This applies to services above, or equal to, a specific level on the hospital procedures classification list. It is also available from the 31st day of hospitalisation.

- *Financial or physical situation of the patient.* This applies to war pensioners, invalidity pensioners, people injured in workplace accidents and pregnant women. It also applies to handicapped children and adolescents.[28]

The amounts contributed to the social security fund are regarded as fair but also at their peak. Some French people (employers and employees) talk of revolution on the streets if the government attempts to increase employee rates of contribution further. While revolution is clearly an exaggeration, protest would almost certainly ensue.

Reimbursement and Access

The French reimbursement system is characteristically form-based, although the introduction of the credit card-sized *carte vitale* has simplified matters. Traditionally, patients had to obtain prescription and /or treatment forms (*feuilles de soins*) from the medical professional consulted, attaching any *vignettes* (stickers) given to them by a pharmacist. In addition, an annual certificate (*attestation annuelle*) issued by the employer was required and, if appropriate, the certificate of unemployment issued by the local office of the national employment service. To obtain reimbursement, these documents had to be delivered or posted to the local CPAM. Some weeks later, claimants received a detailed statement of the amounts to be reimbursed.[29]

Carte Vitale

The *carte vitale* scheme replaces the old *carte d'assure sociale*. In 1998 more than 1.2 billion *'feuilles de soins'* were submitted for reimbursement. The *carte vitale* aims to remove the need for so much form filling, enabling rapid exchange of information between health professionals and the CPAM. The *carte vitale* is not a means of payment.

However, it does enable fast, secure, and automatic reimbursements. It indicates national insurance rights in electronic form, simplifies reimbursement, and obviates the need for postal communications.

If the doctor is suitably equipped, the patient gives the *carte vitale* to the doctor who then puts it in a machine and generates an electronic form which is completed and sent automatically to the CPAM. The French like their privacy and were concerned about the confidentiality of the personal information stored on the card. However, security is ensured by the need for a second doctors' card—the *Carte Professionnel de Santé* (CPS). The CPS acts as the key to the system. It identifies the doctor and access to patient records may be gained only when both cards are entered into the machine. The information subsequently transmitted can only be read by the CPAM. The personal details held are guarded by the *Committée Nationale d'Information Liberté*, and every card holder has the right to access the details kept on the database.

Unfortunately, despite the fact that by early 1999, 30 million *cartes* had been distributed, for a number of reasons many health professionals were not yet equipped with the necessary gadgetry. Allowing for this eventuality, *cartes vitales* are accompanied by 'low-tech' written proof of entitlement to medical insurance.

Couverture Maladie Universale (CMU)—Universal Health Insurance

In early 1999, the government estimated that up to 25 per cent of the French population delayed medical treatment for financial reasons.[30] Those who did so were the least well-off in society. At the same time, some 3.4 million low-income and unemployed people received medical assistance from local authorities (*l'aide médicale générale*—AMG), and 150,000 people had no medical cover at all—a number of whom had relied on charity.[31] To counter charges of inequity, the government planned without delay to extend medical cover to all those residing in France, including the unemployed. The two-level system which is not linked to employment activity or previous insurance contributions was launched in January 2000 with three guiding principles: simplicity for patients and providers, partnership to ensure mobilisation of all health actors, and the quest for equal rights of access to care.[32]

The first CMU level (CMU *de base*) provides medical coverage to all legal French residents. Those with no existing NHI right are automatically associated to the CNAMTS. The second level (CMU *complémentaire*) provides free supplementary insurance to those earning below FF 3,600 per month for a single person.[33]

Those who previously received RMI or AMG are automatically covered at both levels.[34] Other applicants, after filling out a form to register for the scheme at the local social security office (CPAM), the CMU *complémentaire* beneficiaries can opt for their supplementary cover to be managed by either the local *sécu* on behalf of the CNAMTS, or a supplementary insurer—a *mutuelle*, a provident society, or an insurance company. These organisations pay the physicians directly. Once granted, the right to free treatment is valid for one year, after which needs are re-assessed.

Those covered simply take their proof of qualification to the doctor or pharmacy. The cover offered includes free medical consultations by a doctor of the patient's choice (except *non-conventionné*), free prescriptions for drugs normally reimbursed by the '*sécu*', free laboratory tests, and exemption from hospital expenses. In most cases CMU will also pay for dental care, prostheses and spectacles. And, in the name of equal access to care, the services offered to those patients are to be of the same quality as those offered to everyone else.

The result is free cover for over a million people, and CMU *assurance complémentaire* for 4.7 million others (September 2000).[35] The government estimates that the number of potential beneficiaries is six million—roughly half of whom are recipients (and their dependants) of the RMI, the rest being on low income.[36]

The cost of this extension to French National Health Insurance was estimated at FF 9 billion per year. To cover these costs, a national fund has been established by a contribution of FF 7.2 billion, with the rest coming from supplementary insurers. Those supplementary insurers that take on CMU beneficiaries are given FF 1,500 per applicant. The same amount per person per year is given by the government to the CNAMTS, for those it provides with free supplementary cover.[37]

Providers

Choice

Complete freedom of choice of physician and health service provider is an element that sets the French system apart from its social insurance-based neighbour, Germany.[38] The French are completely free to use any doctor or hospital they wish. They may go directly to a specialist either outside or within a hospital. They can choose public or private care. And they can opt for a standard 'office-based' generalist, a 'family' doctor (simply a generalist to whom they have some loyalty) or a 'referring' doctor. Physicians are only permitted to advertise in the yellow pages and, in a system that promotes direct competition between health-care professionals, business is generated primarily by reputation which is spread by word of mouth. However, health organisations can advertise, and there are adverts for private *conventionné* health centres in the Paris metro. It is obligatory, however, for all practising doctors to display their prices.

Patients take into account a variety of factors when choosing a doctor or hospital, including courtesy, length of appointment, waiting times, cleanliness, catering, and privacy. Interpersonal relations between doctors and patients are very good and highly professional. It is now rare to find evidence of paternalism among generalists, while specialists (traditionally more aloof, perhaps owing to the nature of their work) are increasingly more approachable. They are aware that many patients seek a second opinion.

As a rule, appointments with GPs are between 15 and 30 minutes long. One doctor we spoke to said that she would feel guilty taking money from a patient after a workmanlike

3-5 minute appointment because, owing to fee-for-service provision, there is a real sense that the customer is purchasing a service. In the UK consultations typically take 5-7 minutes.

The degree of choice varies because the dispersal of doctors across France is uneven.[39] In a rural area it is possible that it would be more difficult to change doctor, whereas in towns there is invariably a good range of competing providers. Choice of hospital could be expected in towns and cities.

Primary Care

In 1980, the contract between private physicians and the national insurance system changed. As a consequence, the French primary care sector is divided between sector 1 and sector 2 *conventionné* physicians, and a very small number of *non-conventionné* physicians—sometimes called sector 3. At the end of 1997, 99.6 per cent of physicians were in either sector 1 or 2. Of these, 74 per cent were in sector 1— 83 per cent of GPs and 62 per cent of specialists.[40] Sector 1 practitioners are contracted with the NHI agencies and are paid by fee-for-service according to a nationally negotiated fee schedule (NGAP). The schedule contains a frequently revised relative value scale for medical procedures, negotiated annually between representatives of the government, the sickness funds, and the medical profession. By accepting the fee scale, sector 1 physicians are entitled to certain pension and sickness benefits.[41]

Sector 2 doctors can set their own fees which may exceed the official fee schedule—the excess being covered by the patient. They do not have access to pension or sickness benefits. This sector proved popular, particularly among specialists—only 57 applied the negotiated fees in 1990.[42] As a result, access to this sector has been restricted at various times in recent years—shifting by physicians from sector 1 to sector 2 is no longer permitted.

Of the 175,000 qualified doctors in January 1998 (three per 1,000 inhabitants) 51 per cent were specialists, and 49 per cent GPs. Seventy-five per cent of GPs and 68 per cent of specialists were in private practice.[43]

Liberal generalists are found in *cabinets libéraux*. In organisational terms, *cabinets libéraux* are generally small units of one physician, one assistant, and one secretary. They can be 'individuals' or groups of healthcare professionals. Group practices are more common in large urban areas than in rural areas, where single-person practices dominate. Consultations with all sector 1 *conventionné* specialists currently cost FF 115 (about £11).

As the name suggests, *médecins de famille* (MdF) are generalists who deal with the healthcare requirements of families. Not really a separate group, these doctors know a family history well and patients have a long relationship of fidelity to that doctor. The decision to attend an MdF is that of the patient, and having visited a *médecin de famille*, the patient is not prevented from seeing other generalist doctors.

Patients are free to consult a private practice specialist or ask for an appointment with a hospital-based specialist without being referred by a GP. Those private specialists can continue to treat their patients when they are hospitalised.[44] The standard fee to see a specialist is FF 150 (about £15),[45] but physicians in certain specialties can and do charge significantly more. We came across charges by *conventionné* (sector 2) specialists of up to FF 700 (about £70) per consultation.

Médecins Référent

Efforts have been made to restrict choices available to patients. As part of a sustained programme of patient 'responsibilisation', one key aim has been to reduce cases of 'medical-nomadism' by creating incentives to visit a GP before a specialist.[46] It is claimed that such a system will encourage a more holistic and co-ordinated approach to health care, thereby avoiding incompatible prescriptions and cutting the overall number of visits to physicians.

The system works as follows: patients agree to visit a specific GP as their first contact. If that doctor deems it necessary, he or she will refer the patient to specialists drawn from a pre-determined list. As part of a national campaign to limit pharmaceutical expenditure, *médecins référent* are also obliged to prescribe a certain percentage (ten per cent) of generic drugs.

In compensation for removal of choice, the payment system is reminiscent of the *tiers payant* scheme under which the patient only pays the doctor the portion of the standard list fee (*tarif conventionné*) that would not be reimbursed by the social security, that is FF 34.50 (about £3.50). The CPAM then sends the doctor the remaining FF 80 (about £8). GPs who opt to join the scheme receive FF 150 for each new patient that they take on.

This system is clearly related to the UK system of gatekeeper GPs, and to some US HMOs, and while the proposals were accepted by one general practitioners' union, other generalist and specialist unions fiercely objected to the idea and proposed strikes. Most generalists were reluctant because of the fear that they may be subject to still greater control by the health insurance system and because the detailed patient records they are obliged to keep take up a great deal of time that would be better spent treating patients.[47] Meanwhile specialists objected because of the obvious threat to their incomes if patients were not subsequently referred to them. They argued that patient choice must be preserved. By the end of 1998, only 13 per cent of French generalists had joined the *référent* scheme.[48] An OECD study suggests that this limited take-up by physicians is owing to the limited financial incentives.[49]

Municipal Medical Centres

Aside from liberal generalists and specialists, there are also estimated to be between 1,000 and 2,000 municipal centres where salaried doctors provide primary and preventive care. They are operated by municipalities, mutual benefit organisations, trade unions, the Red Cross, and other groups and play an important role in providing services for the poor.[50]

These centres, aimed at the disadvantaged in the locality, were obliged to treat all people, insured or otherwise. Prices are the same as those set nationally for the primary sector.

The long-term effect of CMU on the financing of these organisations is not yet clear. Presumably, those who benefit will either continue to attend the municipal centre, or will feel able to go to a *conventionné* doctor.

Hospital Services: Consumer Choice of Hospital

Hospitals in France are of three types: public, private profit-making, and private non-profit making. Almost two-thirds of all hospital beds are in public hospitals.

Public hospitals: These tend to be larger than private hospitals, are generally well-equipped and provide facilities for research and training of medical students. Public hospitals in France were given managerial autonomy by the Hospital Law in 1991.[51] In 2000, there were roughly 1,050 public health establishments with 323,098 beds (5.5 per 1000 population—1998 figures) The main types were:

- Regional hospitals. Large organisations usually based in cities with university medical schools. There are 29 such hospitals, some of which are composed of many smaller hospitals.

- Hospital Centres. These are found in *Départment* capitals. Many provide specialised care for certain conditions such as mental illness or cancer.

- Local Hospitals. They provide basic care and are not as well equipped as regional hospitals.[52]

Private non-profit hospitals: These typically deal with medium- to long-term care. They have the same obligations as public hospitals, follow the same rules of operation, and financing, except those regarding the employment of staff. They include around twenty specialist cancer centres. In 1998, this sector had 24,782 beds.

Private for-profit hospitals: They concentrate on acute care and particularly surgery. There are many small establishments, although there has been a recent move towards concentration. This sector represents 20 per cent of the total hospital capacity. In 1998, there were 98,813 for-profit hospital beds in France.

In 1998, 1.2 million people were employed in French hospitals. However, France has a lower number of hospital-based specialists than Germany, Sweden, the UK, and Italy. Public hospitals are subject to tight budget controls and doctors are salaried. Specialists in private hospitals are normally paid on a fee-for-service basis and are free to run their clinics as they believe best. Consequently, France has had to rely on foreign doctors to fill many unwanted public-sector posts.

However, public hospitals are perceived to be technically capable and responsive to consumers, and so many people feel there is no *need* to use private hospitals as in Britain merely in order to get quick treatment. Perhaps because of this, there is less ideological suspicion of private sector healthcare providers in France.

The level of funding in public hospitals is determined by the government. As a cost cutting measure, since 1984, public and private hospitals which participate in the NHI schemes have been financed under a global budget based on the previous year's expenditure.[53] Since 1996, regional hospital associations (ARH) have been responsible for allocating funds to individual hospitals on the basis of an overall regional budget. Negotiated contracts take into account the relative health costs and activity level and last for three to five years. They also outline development programmes on the basis of the General Regional Health Organisation Plans (*Schéma régionale d'organisation sanitaire*—SROS). Funding is through the reimbursement of services *per diem*—though there are also attempts to adopt diagnosis related groups (DRGs).[54]

Although there is no fixed budget for private hospitals, regional agencies sign contracts with them. These contracts outline activity levels and specify spending targets.[55] The payment of providers in private hospitals and private practice is largely set by the NHI regime. Profit-making hospitals are funded by a combination of *per-diem* fees and fee-for-service within a global budget.[56]

When judging hospitals, consumers considered cleanliness, decor and so on to be secondary to excellence of treatment provided. On the other hand, privacy, high quality food and access to bottled water are almost taken for granted. The suggestion that hospital care would be based in a room of more than two patients, let alone a mixed ward, elicited horror from the patients we spoke to.

Union representation: Only about 40 per cent of doctors in France are trade union members. Moreover, membership is highly fragmented along occupational, geographical and ideological lines. Three principal unions represent both generalists and specialists in private practice: the *Conféd-ération des Syndicats Médicaux Français* (CSMF), the *Fédération des Médecins de France* (FMF), and *Médecins généralistes de France* (MG France). Learned societies, of which there are a wide variety and whose principal purpose is to promote and discuss scientific advances in medicine, also play a lobbying role.[57] The relative splintering of physicians in France weakens the power of doctors against the state, but they make up for their organisational weakness by resorting to direct action, typically including demonstrations and collective withdrawal from administrative tasks.[58]

The regional unions of doctors, created in 1993, were designed to improve management of the health system. Made up of members of the profession, they constitute the interface between doctors and public decision-makers.

Emergency Services

There are two emergency services available to the French—except for Parisians who have four. The two main services are:

- *Pompiers-médicaux:* These are specially trained 'fire-fighters/first-aiders' and are not qualified to deal with complicated problems

- *Service d'Aide Médicale Urgente* (SAMU): This service is the pride and joy of the French. Having taken the patient's details and symptoms, the operator will put callers through to the doctor on call (*de permanence*). According to his diagnosis, arrangements will be made for a doctor and/or ambulance team to be sent to administer first aid and, if necessary, take the patient to hospital. The basic fee is FF 2,500 per hour. If patients are not part of the social security scheme they must pay the whole fee. If patients are hospitalised, they pay nothing (*prise en charge*), but if the patient is not hospitalised, he or she must pay 30 per cent—which may be partially reimbursed by a *mutuelle* if the patient is a member of one.

Pharmacies, Pharmaceuticals and Laboratories

Seemingly ubiquitous, pharmacies are usually the first port of call for ailing French people. In addition to pharmaceutical products, they also provide general advice about local health services, including lists of doctors and hospitals.

The sickness funds only reimburse the cost of products prescribed by a doctor, not ease or comfort drugs such as vitamins. Reimbursement is either at 35 per cent (denoted by a blue sticker on the pack), or 65 per cent (a white sticker). However, for vital or costly drugs and those for serious conditions, full reimbursement may be made.[59]

As discussed above, it is possible to have the relevant part of the cost paid directly by the sickness fund, in which case, the patient only pays the chemist the percentage not covered.

In addition to national control through the *Objectif National des Dépenses d'Assurance-Maladie* (ONDAM), the pharmaceutical industry in France is bound by the Pharmaceutical Sector Agreement and by complex procedures necessary to gain approval for reimbursement. These involve drug evaluation by the *Commission de la Transparence* and price regulation by the Economic Committee.

The sector agreement has an appendix that lists the permitted rates of growth by therapeutic class. Companies can either negotiate and sign a 'convention' agreement with the Economic Committee or have their drug prices fixed (probably reduced) by public decree. If sales exceed the target, companies have to make penalty payments covering at least 25 per cent of the excess. It means that companies can be punished for selling too much of a product. These penalties are called 'quantity discounts for everybody'.

ONDAM specifies the 'envelope' of total healthcare expenditure, which, in accordance with an annually reviewed law of social security finance (*Loi de Financement pour la Sécurité Sociale*) must not grow by more than a specified percentage. The 2000 ONDAM was 2.5 per cent above the 1999 total. The total amount is divided into sub-sections for hospitals, ambulatory care, pharmaceuticals and numerous other healthcare goods and services. Each of these sectors is threatened with penalty payments if they fail to adhere to the target.[60]

Laboratoires

Patients take their prescription stating the need for a test (blood, urine, saliva, etc.) to private medical laboratories. Found on most high streets, laboratories look like a cross between a surgery and a pharmacy—they all have a blue cross logo. Patients are tested, given the test results, and pay. Results are not sent direct to a doctor as this would restrict the patient's choice.

Public Health

French public health schemes are planned and designed at ministry level and then implemented, publicised and monitored by the CRAM and CPAM. Schemes to reduce smoking, alcoholism, drug addiction, the incidence of AIDs, and accidents both at home and in the workplace, are common.

Health Service Reforms

As a proportion of GDP, healthcare expenditure was 4.2 per cent in 1960, and rose to a peak of 9.8 per cent in 1993-1995. In 1998 it was 9.7 per cent.[61] During the 1960s and early 1970s, steep rises in health expenditure did not seem to pose a problem. At a time of national growth, it was logical to devote an increasing tranche of national wealth to areas of unsatisfied yet important need—and this pattern is seen around the developed world. Annual increases were between six and 14 per cent.[62] The first oil crisis of 1973 briefly interrupted this trend, but in subsequent years health expenditure saw sustained growth in real terms even though national economic growth was clearly slowing. In recent years successive French governments have been preoccupied with cost-cutting.

The French demand and receive more healthcare services than any other European population. For example, in its annual household survey in 1998, *CREDES* 'reported on a sample of 23,035 persons, representative of 95 per cent of households in France.[63] The report concluded that during one month, 33 per cent of interviewees had visited a doctor 'at least once'; 19 per cent visited a GP; eight per cent a specialist; and six per cent visited both—'at least once'.[64]

Reforms designed to stabilise welfare budgets were largely introduced by the ubiquitous ministerial plans. Such 'plans' have been introduced roughly every 18 months since 1975.[65] Three methods have been used. First, governments have tried to increase revenue by raising levels of employee and employer contribution. Second, they have tried to reduce reimbursement levels or the scope of reimbursement. This option was used by the majority of *plans de rédressement* effected between 1976 and 1993, to successfully move to a higher level of co-payment for primary care benefits, and to a level of public finance lower than 60 per cent by 1997.[66] Third, some French administrations sought to finance the deficits by borrowing. The Juppé reforms set out to consolidate the social security debt and increase the period of debt repayment. Such a strategy is clearly not sustainable in the long term.[67]

Reform in France initially focused on public hospitals.[68] The introduction of global budgeting (mentioned above) for hospitals appears to have been partially successful in limiting growth in expenditure. More recently, despite ardent opposition by the public and, of course, the highly independent medical profession, primary care has also become a target for government reformers. Plans issued were designed to curb spending in primary care by setting national targets with collective and individual sanctions for overshoot, and by linking doctors' fees with the levels of prescriptions and overall spending.

From 1994 mandatory practice guidelines (*Références Médicales Opposables*—RMOs), were introduced as a means of cost containment and of standardising patient care—a form of health services provision audit. Those doctors who did not comply could be fined up to £2,000, and, in 1996, 186 were investigated and 75 were fined.[69] However, this proposal to impose fines was overturned as unconstitutional in late 1998 by the constitutional court, because it was a collective sanction that penalised doctors who had not exceeded the budget.[70]

Despite dislike for what doctors saw as 'rationing', the RMOs led to a situation in the spring of 1998 when, having remained within their health spending budget for the previous financial year, French GPs were given a 'bonus' of about £930. Writing in the *British Medical Journal*, Dorozynski comments that:

> many doctors protested ...[that] the principle of a bonus was unethical because a doctor should not be rewarded for prescribing less. Others, including some of the medical associations, termed the bonus a 'poisoned gift', arguing that accepting it was tantamount to accepting the principle of controlled health expenditures—rationing.[71]

Summary

French health care is an example of a system based on a mixture of public and private provision and finance. Apart from those entitled to free cover because of low income, the vast majority of the French pay for health care in three main ways. Their main system is a cross between a social insurance scheme and a hypothecated tax, and recently has become more like a hypothecated tax. In addition the French also pay voluntary supplementary insurance premiums and make out-of-pocket payments. Their awareness of the high cost has made them demanding customers.

Provision is also a mixture of central control and almost anarchic independence. French governments have been very concerned about rising costs. Salaried doctors in public hospitals are indifferent to the price of services because their incomes are independent of their activities, and consequently public hospitals have been subject to tight budgets and heavy controls. However, there is a significant private hospital sector and a substantial number of specialist doctors are fiercely independent. The end result is that French people have as free a choice of doctor or hospital as anywhere in the world.

3

Germany: The System

Political and Administrative Structures

Unlike France, Germany has a federal system of government and a political culture concerned since Nazi times with avoiding the over-concentration of power. German reunification took place in October 1990, following the fall of the Berlin Wall in 1989, and there are now 16 *Länder*, five of which comprised the former East Germany. Each *Land* has its own elected parliament (*Landtag*) which appoints the *Land* government, its own administrative authorities and an independent judiciary. All *Länder* have ministries of social security and most have health ministries.

The chancellor is the executive head of the federal government. The legislative branch of government is bicameral, consisting of the Federal Assembly (*Bundestag*) and the Federal Council (*Bundesrat*). There are no elections for the *Bundesrat*. Instead, *Länder* governments are directly represented by members wielding votes (from three to six) proportionate to population size.[1]

Social Insurance

The German system of social insurance was first established on the national level in 1883 by Bismarck. Three founding principles are commonly identified: solidarity, subsidiarity, and corporatism.[2] When Germans speak of solidarity, they mean that the government takes responsibility for ensuring universal access and that everybody contributes according to their means. It does not imply public sector monopoly, as it does in the UK.

Subsidiarity suggests a decentralised system under which policy is implemented by the smallest feasible political and administrative units in society. This doctrine is endorsed by political parties of all persuasions and is embedded in the German constitution—the Basic Law of 1949. In health care, subsidiarity means that the government is only responsible for setting the legislative framework and establishing the corporatist bargaining process.

Corporatism is seen in the democratically elected representation of employees and employers on the governing boards of sickness funds and in the importance of national and regional decision-making bodies which negotiate the terms of medical care and reflect the interests of groups such as doctors, dentists, pharmacists, the pharmaceutical industry, and insurers.[3] The result is that it is difficult for any one group to change the rules, or to raise fees or contribution rates without the consent of the other parties.[4]

The Federal Chamber of Physicians and the Federal Chamber of Dentists are responsible for deciding on access to medical and dental practice in general, licensing doctors and dentists, and setting standards for medical practice. They interpret the code of professional ethics and have increasingly come under pressure to address quality assurance more vigorously than they have in the past.[5]

The federal government stipulates what is to be contained in the comprehensive package of benefits covered by the self-administered structures of the system. Alongside the public facilities at local and federal level, other key bodies in health services provision include the national associations of insurance providers (statutory and private health insurance), associations of physicians and dentists in primary care, the chamber of independent health professions, hospital associations and the charity associations.[6]

The ministries in each *Land* are responsible for passing their own laws, supervising subordinate authorities, and financing investment in the hospital sector. The *Länder* are subdivided into administrative districts and local authorities (towns, municipalities, counties) all of which have numerous competencies in the healthcare system.[7]

Finance

Health care is financed by a combination of statutory health insurance, general taxation, private health insurance, and some user co-payments. At 10.3 per cent of GDP (1997), total expenditure on health care is high by European standards. In 1998 around 60 per cent of funding was derived from compulsory and voluntary contributions to statutory health insurance, about 21 per cent from general taxation and 11 per cent from patient payments. Private insurance (see p. 61) accounted for the remaining seven per cent.[8]

Health insurance is one of the four branches of the social security system.[9] The others are accident insurance, retirement insurance, and unemployment insurance. Membership of the *Gesetzliche Krankenversicherung* (GKV) system is compulsory for the vast majority of Germans. Only those who earn above the national insurance threshold may choose whether or not to pay contributions.[10]

Those subject to compulsory sickness insurance include:

- Employed people earning beneath a certain threshold, as well as people receiving vocational training.

- Unemployed persons receiving benefits from the Federal Labour Administration. The unemployed and their dependants are protected by a federal law that requires sickness funds to provide the same benefits for the unemployed as for the employed. Premiums are paid for two-thirds of the unemployed, but the remainder receive care outside the GKV system through local social welfare agencies—*Sozialamt* (see p. 64).

- Students, trainees, artists and publicists.

- Pensioners and pension claimants who have made the necessary national insurance payments.[11]

Originally, local mutual aid societies, funded by members and, in some cases, employers, were the basis of national health insurance, but the modern system is financed through equal employer-employee contributions. This reliance on income-based premiums for healthcare financing means that wealthy individuals pay more than the less well-off.[12] Like the French, their direct involvement in payment has made the Germans demanding customers and explains why they enjoy some of the best health care in the world.

Once employment commences, the employer registers the worker for social security, firstly with the sickness insurance fund (*Krankenkasse*). The *Krankenkasse* then informs the competent pension and unemployment insurance bodies and sends each person a credit-card-style membership card or *Chip-karte*. This has to be presented to the receptionist at the doctor's or dentist's surgery.[13]

Although a small part of GKV insurers' income comes from public funds, the vast majority comes from member contributions.[14] The funds function as third-party payers, with patients obtaining benefits in kind from providers who are then paid, via one of the 23 local associations of doctors, by the insurer. Unlike in France, Germans do not normally pay doctors' bills.[15]

Contribution levels are determined solely as a percentage of pre-tax income up to the national insurance limit, which is fixed each year. The income limit in 2001 was DM 6,525 in both the old and new *Länder*. In calculating the national insurance threshold, income from gainful employment is counted but family allowances and irregular income—such as overtime (unless predictable and monthly)—are not.

The contributions are not small. In 1993, rates of *GKV* contribution ranged from 8.5 per cent to almost 17 per cent.[16] In 1998 the average contribution rate was 13.5 per cent in the old *Länder* and 13.9 in the new.[17] Half is paid monthly by employer and employee so that if the contribution rate is 13.5 per cent the employee pays 6.75 per cent. For people with earnings below DM 630 per month, only employers have to pay contributions (at a rate of ten per cent for all funds). There is an additional contribution for long-term care insurance (*Pfelgeversicherung*) of 1.7 per cent (1996).[18]

Choice of Fund

Germans are free to choose their insurer, and 'open' sickness funds must accept any applicant.[19] Prior to 1995, the majority of Germans were assigned by law to specific insurance funds. Now, all of those insured under the GKV system (wage earners or salaried employees and the unemployed) are placed on the same footing.[20] Although the government has set out to increase competition, advertising expenditures are restricted to DM 6 (about £2) per insured person per year.[21]

Sickness funds fall into seven groups:

- *Allgemeine Ortskrankenkassen* (General regional funds), known as AOK. Their federal association is in Bonn. AOK is Germany's largest health insurance organisation, covering about 40 per cent of the insured. Traditionally, these local funds tended to be the insurers of last resort, because they were obliged to insure those who did not belong to a particular employer group.

- 13 substitute funds known as *Ersatzkassen*. Their predecessors were the early mutual aid societies, and they now cover nearly one-third of the population—until recently, primarily white-collar workers. *Ersatzkassen* are often cheaper than AOK, but AOK has more branches.

- 359 company-based funds known as *Betriebskrankenkassen* (BKK).

- 42 guild funds or *Innungskrankenkassen* (IKK).

- 20 farmers funds or *Landwirtschaftliche Krankenkassen* (LKK).

- One miners' fund known as *Bundesknappschaft*.

- One sailors' fund known as *See-Krankenkasse*.[22]

There are seven associations of sickness funds, all of which are self-administered corporate bodies subject to state supervision.[23] Sickness fund boards are usually made up of equal number of employers and employees, although the *Ersatzkassen* boards represent members only.

Having joined an insurer, members subsequently have the freedom to change insurer once per year—the final deadline for cancellation is 30 September. The cancellation only becomes effective if the employer has been presented with a membership card from another health insurance company before 31 December. It is also possible to change insurer upon moving to a new employer.

Free choice of insurer became effective for most fund members at the beginning of 1997. Sickness funds are free to set their own contribution rates, but some commentators have argued that price competition is not possible since the sickness funds have to offer (almost) the same benefits for very similar contribution rates.[24]

However, users are moving to funds with lower premiums. Between 1995 and 1997 the membership of the AOK general local funds fell by four per cent because its contribution rate was one of the highest.[25] The AOKs lost 479,000 members in 1997, 400,000 in 1998 and 292,000 in 1999 while the BKKs increased their membership by 335,000, 516,000 and 971,000 respectively.[26]

The most notable result of competition has been the marked reduction in the number of sickness fund insurers due to mergers. The total number of funds fell from 1,200 in 1985, to 453 in 1998. The number of local funds (AOK's), the 'insurers of last resort', fell even more dramatically from around 270 in 1992 to 17 in 1999.[27]

Equalisation of Risks Mechanism[28]

It became apparent to the government that certain funds were in increasing financial difficulty because they insured lower-income and higher-risk groups.[29] By recruiting higher-income Germans and foreign residents, some funds had been able to increase their revenues substantially.[30] However, *Krankenkasse* are under an obligation to break even and some faced the choice of either restricting benefits or raising premiums. Initially, the employer-employee controlled boards raised premiums and offered more comprehensive services than those mandated by federal law in order to compete with the substitute funds and private health insurers for higher-income groups.[31] However, rising premiums had a major impact on the competitiveness of German industry, and to counteract the effects of unequal member demographics, an equalising pool mechanism was introduced in two stages in 1994 and 1995 (prior to the 1996

liberalisation of funds) to assist funds with a disproportion-
ate number of high-risk groups, especially the elderly and
chronically ill, and to limit risk selection (or 'cream-skim-
ming') as much as possible.[32] Payment into and out of the
pool is based on a complex calculation, undertaken by the
Federal Agency for Insurance, based on age, gender, and
the number of disabled pensioners. The mechanism as it
stands is subject to criticism, some parties arguing that it
is anti-competitive, while others suggest it needs to be more
sensitive to avoid risk selection.[33]

Package of Benefits In Kind

Having joined a sickness fund, the right to medical benefits
and services is independent of the size of contribution.[34] The
health insurance fund pays the cost of medical and dental
treatment, drugs and medicines. Statutory health insurance
also covers prevention, early detection and treatment of
disease; medical rehabilitation; payment of sickness
benefits; pregnancy and maternity benefits; and health
promotion.[35]

The sickness fund normally assumes financial responsibility for the cost of spectacles and other aids and appli-
ances up to a fixed maximum, although prior approval is
required. Under certain conditions, travelling costs may
also be partially or wholly paid by the sickness fund.

Members of an employee's family are also covered,
usually spouse and children up to the age of 18. If children
are not pursuing any gainful activity, they are covered up
to the age of 23 or, if they are in vocational training or
studying, up to the age of 25, providing they do not have an
income in excess of a set limit (DM 640 [about £213] per
month in 2000).[36]

Eligibility for coverage is portable throughout the
country.[37] Registration at doctors' offices, hospitals, and
specialised facilities takes only a few minutes, and individuals are then able to receive medical attention without
delay. In 1993, *Chip-karten* (smart cards) replaced an
insurance certificate (*Krankenschein*) system, that had
served as identification and membership card for 100 years.

Public Health and Preventive Health Care

According to one government estimate in 1997, only four per cent of the population had a thoroughly healthy lifestyle.[38] There are problems related to smoking, diet and lack of exercise. Numerous federal and state institutions, as well as private non-profit organisations, provide information, courses and advice on health matters. The statutory health insurers focus their efforts on:

- *Preventive check-ups during pregnancy*. Insured women are entitled to ten medical examinations during pregnancy to monitor the health of mother and child.

- *Early detection examinations for children*. Provision is made for ten examinations at various ages.

- *Health check-ups*. Starting at the age of 35, all insured persons can undergo an examination every two years, during which their doctor checks especially for signs of major illnesses characteristic of developed societies such as heart and circulatory disorders, kidney disease and diabetes.

- *Preventive cancer check-ups*. Insured persons are entitled to an annual examination for early detection of cancer. For women these examinations begin at the age of 20, and for men at the age of 45.

- *Preventive dental care for children and young people*. Together with kindergartens and schools, the health insurers conduct action programmes for the prevention of dental problems that target children up to the age of 12. In addition, children and young people between the ages of six and 18 can have a personal dental check-up every six months.[39]

Members are also entitled to domestic nursing care where it is not possible to hospitalise patients. Patients with children under the age of 12, or who are handicapped, and who cannot be looked after by another person at home, may also receive domestic help.

Direct Payment by Patients

Although German co-payments have risen recently, they remain modest by international standards and have not been a major tool of cost containment. Most patients do not pay for doctors' bills and care remains almost free at the point of delivery.[40] The following are the main co-payments:

- Prescription fees which vary with the size of the prescription package but are not more than the cost of the product (small: DM 9 [about £3]; medium: DM 11 [about £3.50]; and large: DM 13 [about £4.20]). Vitamins and medicines taken for certain illnesses such as the common cold or influenza must be paid for in full

- Dressings, at a flat rate of DM 9 (about £3.00) per prescription, though not more than the cost of the product

- Bandages, inserts and aids for compression therapy, at 20 per cent of cost

- Hospital hotel expenses daily charge (DM 17 per day [about £5.50] in the West, and DM 14 [about £4.50] in the East), for the first 14 days

- In-patient preventive and rehabilitation care (DM 25 [about £8] per day in the West and DM 20 [about £6.40] in the East) for the first 14 days

- Travel expenses (DM 25 [about £8.30] for each medically necessary journey).[41]

The same low co-payment levels do not apply to the provision of dental services where there are up to 100 per cent co-payments for some procedures especially for prosthetic services. Standard fees charged by dental technicians and dentists for dentures and crowns are reimbursed by the sickness fund up to 50 per cent of approved rates. This refund percentage can be increased by a further ten per cent if you undergo a check-up every year.

There are significant exemptions from co-payment. Children are exempt (except for dentures and travel), along with individuals injured while at work, pregnant women and war victims. So too are recipients of educational assistance, unemployment allowances, benefits promoting vocational training or employment, as well as insured people whose monthly family income does not exceed the following limits: singles DM 1,764 (about £570); first dependant DM 2,425 (about £780); each additional dependant DM 441 (about £140). The chronically ill are exempt from contributions towards the cost of prescription drugs, bandages and dressings and towards the cost of travel if they have had to spend one per cent of their income on treatment of the same illness over the last year.[42]

According to Busse and Howorth, the exemptions to co-payment affect about eight million persons and all 12 million insured children.[43] There is also a maximum co-payment for everyone—two per cent of annual taxable income. At the end of each year, payments for drugs, dentistry and hospital care are added up and amounts above the two per cent threshold are reimbursed.[44]

Supplementary Health Insurance

In mid-1999 there were 453 statutory sickness funds with about 72 million insured persons (50.7 million members plus their dependants). As in France, GKV patients may also obtain supplementary cover from the private sector.[45] At the end of 2000, about 7.5 million (more than nine per cent of the population) members of the GKV system had supplementary insurance—double the proportion in 1980. Those who pay for supplementary insurance do so in order to receive treatment in greater privacy, to cover overseas treatment, the hospital daily charge, and to meet co-payments for prescriptions, optical and dental care.[46]

Private Insurance (PKV)

The Bismarckian system of social security was based on the principle that the state should provide only for those unable to provide for themselves, and consequently there was a continuing role for private enterprise alongside the state scheme. Existing mutual assistance bodies were well suited to offering these schemes and, even today, half of the 115 organisations writing private health insurance business are mutual.[47] The others are for-profit insurers. Of these 115 organisations, 51 companies account for 99 per cent of premium income. They operate nationwide and are members of a powerful lobby group, the Association of Private Health Insurers. The remaining 65 are small private associations and local relief funds offering mainly supplementary insurance.

Those earning more than the national insurance threshold of DM 6,525 in 2001 may choose to opt out of GKV and contract with private insurers, and roughly one in three high-income earners do so.[48] In 2000, 7.4 million Germans had comprehensive private insurance.

While the majority of the civil service workforce of seven million are covered by GKV, since the Healthcare Reform Act came into force in 1989, some two million civil servants (*Beamte*) are provided for separately. For these civil servants, plus certain *Freiwilligen* (independent professionals such as lawyers and physicians and the self-employed who, with the exception of farmers and artists are not mandatorily insured in the GKV system), private insurance is the preferred method. Unlike others earning above the national insurance threshold, *Beamte* do not tend to belong to the statutory insurance scheme on a voluntary basis because the government (as the employer) will not pay the usual 50 per cent of the insurance premium.[49]

Beamte are insured against the risks of illness through *Beihilfe* (state assistance) and are reimbursed directly by their employer (federal, state, and local government) up to a proportion (between 50 and 90 per cent) of their healthcare costs. Most of the individuals in this group—which includes teachers, police, and federal railway civil servants —purchase private health insurance to cover the cost of services not reimbursed by the government assistance. *Beamte* civil servants have special low tariffs from private insurers because they only pay roughly half the cost of medical care. However, the self-employed can pay high tariffs for health cover because they have no subsidy from an employer.[50]

With the above exceptions, irrespective of whether employees are insured under the state or private health insurance, the employer and employee each pay half the premium.[51]

Unlike those for GKV funds, private premiums are related to risk.[52] Hence, subject to some restriction, premiums are based on age, gender, and health status at the time of enrolment, after which premiums are not adjusted for age or medical history.

Private insurance, unlike statutory insurance, enables the insured to tailor their cover to suit their needs. Depending on the policy type, the insured choose between policies which refund costs in full and those which cover only certain elements or a fixed percentage of medical expenses. They can also choose policies with a front-end deductible (or excess), in which case the premiums are significantly reduced. For example, with an annual deductible of DM 1,900 (about £610) the premium paid by a 33-year-old woman for the outpatient element of her insurance cover would amount to about 32 per cent of the full-cover premium.[53]

Those with full private cover make their own arrangements for treatment and receive an invoice that they must settle. However, it is now common for hospital physicians to send treatment invoices directly to the insurer rather than via the patient. The bill is based on an official scale of fees. That scale allows doctors treating private patients a degree of leeway, so much so that charges in the private sector can be more than twice as high as fees charged (by the same physician) to GKV insured patients.[54]

Despite the above choices, the most obvious benefits of private insurance include luxuries such as private rooms and access to treatment by the chief of a hospital department rather than a less senior doctor.[55]

Is the GKV/private insurance split divisive? With the exception of a young vocal minority, the ideological divide between the sectors that we see in Britain is not replicated in Germany. There is no great desire to have private health insurance because the 'public' treatment is perceived as excellent. Moreover, the privately insured are not generally perceived as health pariahs or queue jumpers, because there are no queues to jump.

The Unemployed

Healthcare insurance in Germany is employment-based. Those who have never worked (including asylum seekers, divorced housewives and homeless people (about 1.5 per cent of the population) are not able to join national insurance. Instead, they receive welfare benefits, *Sozialhilfe*, from the local *Sozialamt*. Each claimant is issued with a *Sozialamt Krankenschein*, a booklet with coupons, for every calendar quarter, which entitles the named person to medical treatment during that period. Physicians send an invoice and are paid by the local *Sozialamt* rather than through their normal quarterly submission to the regional physicians' association.

In a few cases, there is a slightly different procedure. Some *Sozialamt* have negotiated special agreements with local insurers (especially AOK) and use their infrastructure to provide services for the uninsured. The quality of care received by these poorest members of society should be the same as that received by ordinary GKV members. However, those with *Sozialamt* cover have to contact the welfare office to obtain prior authorisation of treatment for many more procedures. Thus, speedy access to treatment is less freely available to those on *Sozialhilfe*.

Moreover, free dental care for those on *Sozialhilfe* only covers amalgam fillings; cosmetic treatments are not provided. Patients who want ceramic fillings or any other treatment that is not judged medically necessary must pay personally. With the exception of the daily charge for hospital treatment, co-payment does not apply to those with very low incomes or on social welfare.[56]

Providers

German primary care is clearly separated from secondary care. Primary care doctors have a gate-keeping role in

Germany, but users have direct access to private specialists outside hospitals in local practices, some of whom have access to hospital facilities. An estimated four in ten patients do not go to a GP before seeing a specialist.[57]

Treatment under GKV is provided by doctors or dentists recognised by the sickness funds—more than 90 per cent of established medical practitioners. All physicians practising under GKV must join an association which controls the physician payment system and monitors physician performance. A list of these medical practitioners is available at the local sickness fund offices.

German physician supply is high at 3.4 per 1,000 in 1997 (84,778 of which are GPs—one per 1,000).[58] Indeed, Germany has one of the highest physician/population ratios in the world. Fewer than half of the nation's 181,000 doctors are in private practice. The others work in hospitals or administration or are engaged in research.

Unlike France, there is no quota for medical students because the German constitution guarantees the right to medical education, subject only to entry qualifications. Instead, since the Health Care Reform Act of 1992, the Regional Physicians' Associations have geographically and by speciality restricted the settlement of new doctors.[59] In 1995 there was no *Land* where all sub-regions were open for all specialties. However, there were openings for all specialties somewhere in the federal republic.

The majority of primary physicians operate in a single physician practice. According to Graig (1999), only about one in five physicians are in 'group' practices. Indicating some change, however, Busse puts the figure at around 25 per cent of physicians in 2000.[60]

The utilisation of primary physicians increased considerably between 1988 and 1995, from 5.5 treatment invoices for every GKV member in 1988 to 6.9 in 1995. According to the federal ministry, this increase was mainly due to referrals to specialists, but the number of services also increased. Whereas in the former West Germany, in 1990, 39 services per insured person were provided, in 1995 it was already 53 services.[61]

General Practice

Family practitioners (GPs and physicians without speciali-sation) are chosen by GKV members, ostensibly for a financial quarter.[62] GPs have to complete a five-year course of further training to become a specialist in general medi-cine. The work of a GP in private practice might consist of house calls between 7:30 a.m. and 9:00 a.m., followed by seeing patients at their office until 4:30 p.m. (with two hours for lunch), and then more house calls until 8:00 p.m.[63]

Patients may either telephone a GP for an appointment, or may simply go to the office and wait. Patients must present the doctor of their choice with proof of insurance, usually a sickness insurance *Chip-karte*. In emergencies, however, doctors will treat patients without requiring this card.

Primary Specialists

While using GPs as gatekeepers is encouraged, there is freedom of access to a wide variety of primary private practice specialists.[64] These primary practice specialists provide many of the services that are provided by hospital outpatient departments under the NHS.[65] One might expect to find the following specialists in any medium-sized German town: *Internists, Kinderspezialist* (specialist paediatrician), *Frauenarzt* (gynaecologists), *Augenarzt* (eye specialist), *Hals-Nasen-Ohrenheilkunde* (ear, nose and throat—ENT), *Dermatologe* (dermatologist), *Chirurgin* (surgeon), *Sportmedizin* , *Urologe* (urologist), *Zahnmedizin* (dentist), *Physiologin* (physiologist), *Osteopath* (osteopath). Only a few specialties (psychiatry for example) are poorly represented in some regions. There is strong competition between these physicians, but they are not permitted explicitly to advertise their superiority or denigrate compet-itors.

The training of specialists is long in Germany, and those who wish to practice in the private sector must do at least six years of hospital-based service prior to setting up practice on their own. This is not regarded as a great hardship, as the long-term financial prospects are excellent.

Bridging the Care Divide

Until recently, primary physicians were not able to treat patients in hospitals and hospitals did not provide out-patient surgical and diagnostic services. This separation of responsibilities sometimes led to long referral chains, with inadequate and uncoordinated record keeping. The 1993 Health Care Act tried to tackle the problem by allowing independent GPs and specialists to gain access to a certain number of hospital beds. These external hospital specialists have surgeries of their own, where they typically treat patients, but they may also reserve a number of hospital beds for inpatient treatment. In 1994, six per cent of hospital doctors were external doctors.[66] As part of the same cost cutting and efficiency trend, hospitals are strongly encouraged to perform outpatient surgery and pre- and post-operative care for outpatients.[67]

Payment of Professionals by GKV Patients

Physician incomes are high in comparison to other self-employed or academic professions, averaging DM 184,900 per year in 1998 before tax (about £60,000) and vary significantly between sections of the profession: ENT specialists average DM 250,800 (about £80,500) and GPs DM 155,000 (about £50,000).[68]

Insurers have no direct relationship with providers. They pay regional physicians' associations who pay physicians from a capitated pool. This remuneration must be accepted as payment in full. The sums paid are worked out by using a uniform value scale introduced in 1977. It lists over 2,000 services which can be provided by physicians for remuneration, subject to certain preconditions.[69]

Most of the associations divide the budget into three separate pools (basic, laboratory, and other services). The points of all the physicians in the region are aggregated in these separate pools, and conversion factors applied to each physician to determine their share.[70] Thus, GKV physicians do not know exactly how much they will earn from services to patients. Moreover, when a physician orders extra laboratory tests or treatment for his or her patients, the other physicians in the region, and not the sickness fund, lose income to that physician.[71] A warning system has been introduced to notify physicians who exceed the average by 40 per cent that their fees will be reduced, unless they can convince a panel of physicians and sickness fund representatives that the service was justified. About seven per cent of German physicians receive such notices in a year and about two per cent (about one-third of those receiving notification) have their fees reduced.[72]

Payment of Professionals by Private Patients

Those with private insurance generally pay providers directly and are subsequently reimbursed.

Physicians who opt out of national health insurance and treat only patients with private insurance (a fairly limited number) receive higher payments than their GKV-associated counterparts. Unlike the relative value scales under GKV, specific fees are assigned to about 7,000 items, (listed in a Federal Ministry Ordinance) allowing these physicians to charge up to 3.5 times the sickness fund rates.[73] Both the uniform value scale and the private procedures scale are used by physicians who treat a mixture of private and GKV insured patients.

Hospital Services: Consumer Choice of Hospital

German hospitals are under diverse ownership, which, in an environment where patients choose which hospital to attend, further encourages competition and constant efforts to raise standards. In 1997, in addition to the 2,040 general hospitals (831 public hospitals, 835 hospitals maintained by independent non-profit organisations and 374 private hospitals owned by private companies) with a total of 594,000 beds, there were 229 other hospital facilities or clinics. About 190,000 beds were also available in 1,404 preventive care or rehabilitation centres. This meant that around 50 per cent of hospital beds were in the public sector, about 38 per cent (rising from 35 per cent in 1995), were run by private, non-profit organisations and roughly 12 per cent by private, for-profit institutions.[74] Taking into account all in-patient beds as defined by the OECD, in 1998 there were 762,596 beds—9.3 per thousand population.[75] However, hospital beds are not evenly distributed. In 1992 there were 6.5 beds per 1,000 population in Schleswig-Holstein, but 10.6 in Bremen and 11.0 in Berlin.[76]

Public Hospitals

When a GP considers it necessary to refer a patient to a specialist, polyclinic or similar institution, a referral note (*Uberweisungsschein*) is issued. If hospital treatment is required, except in the case of emergencies, a doctor issues a (*Notwendigkeitsbesheiningung*) certificate stating the patient's need for hospital treatment. The patient sends it to the local sickness fund which in turn issues a form (*Kostenubernahmeschein*) undertaking to cover the costs of treatment in a public ward of a hospital of the patient's choice.[77]

Public hospital-based physicians are salaried employees of the hospital, while their colleagues in private hospitals are paid on a fee-for-service-basis. They are organised in a hierarchical, departmental structure.

Since 1972, dual financing has operated in the German hospital sector: operating costs are met by the sickness funds and capital investment by the *Länder*. Traditionally, payment to hospitals was based on *per-diem* rates that were uniform within a hospital and independent of actual diagnosis, amount of care, or length of stay.[78] The 1993 Health Care Act retained dual finance but introduced a more complex method of reimbursing hospitals which meant they were no longer entitled to full payment of costs.[79] Fixed budgets were calculated for individual hospitals and 1996 saw the introduction of prospective case fees and procedure fees, for a portion of in-patient care.

Towards the end of June 2000, both partners, the German Hospitals' Association (DKG) and the sickness funds, finally agreed to use the Australian AR-DRG system (Australian refined diagnosis related groups) which consists of 661 categories, each with five grades of severity. The new German system will contain between 600 and 800 diagnostic groups and should be introduced in 2003.[80]

Finally, a co-payment for in-patient treatment is applied to all state and private hospital patients. This daily charge (DM 17 [about £5.50]) covers 'hotel' expenses. If patients want more privacy, they may also pay for accommodation in a single or twin-bedded room.

Private Hospitals

Non-profit or community hospitals are typically run by religious orders affiliated with the Catholic or Protestant churches and are partially funded by the German church tax. Private hospitals also receive their capital funds from the state. The physicians who work in the private hospital sector are paid on a fee-for-service-basis.[81]

Voluntary bodies involved in providing health care include among others the *Arbeiterwohlfahrt* (National Association for Workers' Welfare), *Caritas*, the *Deutscher Paritatischer Wohlfahrtsverband* (German Non-Denominational Welfare Association), and the German Red Cross.[82]

Long-term Nursing Care

There has been a greatly increased need for long-term and home care.[83] Any person who is GKV insured is automatically a member of the statutory long-term care insurance (a statutory long-term care fund has been set up within each statutory health insurance fund). Those with private medical insurance must take out private long-term care insurance.

Payment into the German system of long-term care insurance (unlike other such schemes abroad) is funded completely out of equal contributions by employers and employees, currently 1.7 per cent of income.[84]

For non-institutional care, the beneficiary has a choice between benefits in kind (services rendered by one of the long-term care fund's contractual partners, typically a home care agency) and a cash benefit to allow patients to choose the most suitable provision—care by relatives for example.

Although its monetary value is smaller than that of direct service provision—about 70 per cent of the claimants to the insurance scheme applied for cash benefits in Germany (second quarter 1997). In order to meet the needs of individual patients, a combination of the two is also possible.[85]

In Germany the most important service providers of long-term care are private, non-profit organisations. They are usually religious groups or other charitable organisations with a long history of serving the community.

A German Embassy press release (2000) explains that:

> since the plan came into force five years ago after widespread opposition, the number of mobile services available has increased to 13,000 and there are 8,600 permanent institutions on hand to take in people as residents. Meanwhile the number of people needing care at home has more than doubled from 600,000.[86]

According to the health ministry, in 2000, about 1,860,000 people in need of care were receiving monthly help in cash or in kind, 1,310,000 of them at home, 550,000 in institutions.

Pharmaceuticals

Pharmacists are highly qualified in Germany and act as the first point of call for many people. Prescription medicines can be obtained from all dispensing chemists for the same price.[87] In 1995 there were 21,000 public pharmacies in Germany with nearly 40,000 pharmacists in the West and 4,700 in the East, about one for every 4,000 inhabitants —the EU average. Their numbers are not controlled, and they have a monopoly on dispensing prescription-only products.[88]

Ninety four per cent of pharmacy turnover in the West comes from drugs; 62 per cent prescription drugs, 30 per cent over-the-counter drugs and two per cent freely available. Pharmaceutical consumption per head in 1995 was 11.4 prescriptions for men with 355 daily doses on average, and 15.4 prescriptions for women with 496 daily doses— giving an average of 13.5. Of the 31 billion prescribed daily doses in 1995, 57 per cent were prescribed by GPs. By 1997 this figure had fallen slightly to between 55 and 56 per cent.[89]

Control of Pharmaceutical Expenditure

The annual budget for pharmaceutical consumption is fixed by the health insurance funds and the associations of sickness fund doctors. Expenditure is controlled by four methods—a short negative list, reference prices, a pharmaceutical spending cap, and encouragement to use generics. In 1999 generics accounted for 39 per cent of all prescription drugs.[90] The negative list comprises products that are not covered by GKV for users over the age of 18.

Reference pricing was introduced in 1989 for drugs whose patent had expired. Reference prices are administratively fixed reimbursement levels for medicines with similar properties. Individuals who wish to obtain a product priced above the reference level, have to pay the difference between this market price and the official reference price.[91]

Germany is the third largest pharmaceutical market in the world and has some 1,100 pharmaceutical manufacturers.[92] The quality, effectiveness and safety of drugs and medicines are tested in accordance with the state marketing authorisation procedure. Approximately 45,000 marketable drugs are available in Germany—more than in any other European country. Furthermore, a dense distribution network consisting of pharmaceutical manufacturers, wholesalers and pharmacies ensures that people throughout the country have access to the medicines they need.[93] While the manufacturer's drug prices are set according to market conditions, there is federal control over mark-ups by wholesalers. The maximum mark-up varies in inverse proportion to the manufacturer's price.

Providers have been vocal in their fight against prescription reforms. After more than a century of independence, doctors have had their professional judgment challenged by a budget-capping mechanism—and at the same time average physician earnings have fallen recently.

Redwood[94] comments that anecdotal and statistical evidence about the impact of budget-capping differs. News stories and the individual testimony of our interviewees point to some doctors fobbing off their more docile patients with cheap products when a costly innovative prescription drug would have been better. In order to remain within their budgets, physicians sometimes transfer their patients to more expensive hospital and clinic-based care which is not on their budget when drug therapy (included in their budget) would have been at least as effective and cheaper.[95]

Powell and Wessen[96] inform us that the serious press in Germany reported that some patients had been told that their physician had reached the ceiling of total points assigned to each specialty group and would not, therefore, be reimbursed for any additional services. Some of our interviewees reported similar experiences, which led doctors to close (take a holiday) towards the end of each financial quarter. Powell and Wessen add that if patients were willing to pay out of pocket, they could continue to receive services or prescription drugs that were previously available under GKV. A recent study indicates that 12 per cent of patients in the GKV system receive the newest innovative drugs, while 48 per cent of private patients receive them.[97]

The US International Trade Commission reports that 'Strict budgetary controls imposed on German physicians mean that they may not always be in a position to prescribe the products that, in their professional opinion, would best suit their patients' needs'. It concluded that there was evidence of a bias against innovative therapies:

> In some cases only patients who specifically request innovative products may receive them, while those who do not are prescribed older, less effective, medicines that do not improve their quality of life or medical condition as much as innovative medicines would.[98]

Health Service Reforms

After years of successful cost control by international standards, Germany's high healthcare expenditure began to come under strong criticism, exacerbated by the perceived threat of an ageing population, increased public demand for all the best the medical world had to offer, rising costs of advancing medical treatments, and supply-side inefficiency.[99]

Until the late 1980s costs were met by raising employer and employee premiums (*Krankenkassen* have a statutory duty to balance their books). However, in periods of sluggish growth this solution was no longer viable.[100]

There have been three stages of reform over the last fifteen years. One prominent interpreter of the German system, Ulrich,[101] identifies three key principles underlying statutory health insurance (GKV): self-administration (whereby healthcare purchasers and providers operate as self-managing units under public law); social partnership (responsibility for meeting the financial cost is shared between employers and employees); and solidarity (the economically stronger members of society support the weaker).

According to Ulrich, private health insurance systems rely on three different principles: the insurance principle (premiums are risk-related, mainly taking into account age, sex, and the medical history of the insured); the principle of equivalence (whereby the level of contribution reflects the desired level of coverage); and personal precaution (all individuals are responsible for their own health so that premiums may reflect lifestyle variables).[102]

During the 1990s public policies have attempted to move slowly in the direction of the private insurance model, but without abandoning the solidarity still cherished by most Germans.[103]

The first stage led to the 1989 Health Care Reform Act which introduced a reference price system for drugs. Amongst other measures within the Act, certain blue-collar workers became free to change insurer, and a negative list of pharmaceuticals considered to be ineffective was introduced.

The second stage comprised the 1992/3 Health Care Structural Reform Act. The 'Seehofer reform' which came into force in 1993 had two aims: to reduce total healthcare expenditure by ten per cent, and second, to encourage efficiency through greater competition between sickness funds and hospitals.

Graig[104] argues that the most significant feature of the Act was the imposition of separate budget caps on each of the major healthcare sectors: outpatient physicians, hospitals, pharmaceuticals, and dental services. The caps aimed to tie health expenditure to rises in workers' income.

The act targeted the wasteful re-diagnosis of patients moving between sectors by breaking down the barrier between the hospital and primary sectors, chiefly by allowing primary surgery in hospitals.[105]

Competition between GKV sickness funds was encouraged by allowing members to change insurance fund. Moreover, to encourage competition between the sickness funds based on quality of service, not risk selection, the above-mentioned risk equalisation scheme was introduced.[106] Some observers argue that the result has been that sickness funds now compete with other insurance carriers for new members by offering highly variable service packages. Such competition led the press to label funds as 'regular funds', 'superfunds', 'sensational funds', and/or 'five-star funds.' ('*Werr hat das bessere Angebot?*' 1996).[107]

Chip-karten (smart cards) for health insurance purposes were introduced in 1993 to confirm eligibility for coverage. It was also hoped that these smart cards would enhance the coordination of care and improve the flow of information among providers.[108]

The third stage followed in 1996 and 1997. The 1996 Health Insurance Contribution Rate Exoneration Act contained provisions reducing benefits, increasing co-payment levels and also reducing sickness fund contribution rates by 0.4 per cent.[109] The 1996 First and 1997 Second Statutory Health Insurance Restructuring Acts, contained many measures that were subsequently reversed in 1998. Busse[110] comments that policies that were reversed were those which broke 'traditional rules of the system' (uniform availability of benefits, employers and employees sharing contributions equally, provision of services as benefits in kind). One policy to survive was the possibility of new contractual relations between providers and sickness funds.[111] In 1998, the Act to Strengthen Solidarity in Statutory Health Insurance lowered co-payment rates, improved benefits and made balanced financial results possible in 1999.[112]

Most recently, the Reform Act of Statutory Health Insurance 2000 set out to reorganise the health insurance system. These reforms were not budget-cutting measures. Indeed, the government claims that more money will flow into the system each year—roughly DM 4 billion for the year 2000, for example. Instead, the focus is upon changing existing structures so that healthcare supply will be better able to meet the changing demand. In order to strengthen the family doctor system, sickness funds may now offer financial bonuses to those who use GPs as gatekeepers to specialist services. Disputed pharmaceuticals and technologies were removed from the sickness fund's benefits catalogues, while a positive list of reimbursable drugs may now be issued by the *Bundesministerium für Gesundheit*.[113]

Summary

What can we learn? In Germany insurance provides a connection between the people who go out to work and earn their keep and the resources available to healthcare providers. Our reliance on taxation makes it impossible for us to judge whether or not we are receiving value for money. The majority of the population who pay their national insurance contributions accept that they must also pay for the poor, but there is no expectation that in order to ensure access for all there must also be public sector monopoly. On the contrary, the Germans have successfully combined consumer choice and universal access. It is true that the rich can always buy a premium service. They can and do in the UK. But German policy makers do not waste their time trying to stop some people from ever getting more than anyone else. They focus on ensuring that the standard of care available to the poorest people is acceptably high.

4

Lessons for the UK

Is Health Care Different?

For the last 50 years public debate about the NHS has been dominated by the moral imperative that no one should be denied medical care. It has been taken for granted that the NHS is the best method of achieving that aim. We will argue that the evidence from France and Germany is that there are better methods, but first it is necessary to disentangle the questions raised by the apparently unimpeachable moral claim that everyone should have access to health care.

Its main appeal rests on an analogy with emergency situations. If someone is so badly hurt, perhaps bleeding heavily or unable to breathe, any moral system would enjoin any person to offer assistance. Two main concerns arise. First, even if we are speaking only of health care which is an urgent necessity, is public sector monopoly the most effective method of providing it? And second, it must be acknowledged that not all health care is urgent and that a good deal of the expenditure in a prosperous society is on the comfort and convenience of patients. That is, health care has a dual character: it is often a matter of urgent necessity, but much also resembles other consumer goods.

These complications make it very difficult to decide how to define how much health care the government should provide as of right. Writers have spoken of a civilised or decent minimum, core services, basic services, reasonable standards and so on. Some duck the issue altogether by insisting that access should be 'comprehensive', even though no one with practical knowledge of the NHS truly believes that any such goal is possible.

The intractable problem of defining how much care government should guarantee individual members of society is
related to a further complexity. Commentators who seek to
be realistic and to define the 'minimum' or the 'core' come
under attack for accepting inequality of access. The most
extreme version of this theory demands that no one should
ever get more than anyone else, an objective which can only
be approached if the whole national system is under central
control. Yet equality in the sense of uniformity remains the
NHS objective, despite the fact that it has never been the
reality and only a few diehards believe it to be achievable.
All this is quite apart from the unintended consequences of
central direction intended to create a uniform pattern of
care—perhaps the most serious of which is the suppression
of diversity and competition, the chief means by which
progress and learning from the experience of others is
facilitated.

There is a further difficulty, namely that medical need is
not clear-cut. Many systematic studies have found that
well-respected doctors often disagree about both the
diagnosis and the appropriate treatment. This creates the
potential for them to be influenced by financial consider-
ations when there are clinical grey areas. Consequently,
under fee-for-service systems there is a potential for doctors
to carry out unnecessary operations; and when they receive
a fixed salary regardless of the number of patients treated
or the quality of care provided, there is a potential for
under-treatment.

Before governments took responsibility for the poor it was
generally accepted that health care was not exactly like
other consumer goods. Just as a decent human being would
not let someone else starve, so too they would not be allowed
to die or suffer through a lack of health care. The provision
of medical care has always had this moral dimension.
Before it became a government responsibility doctors
provided free care for the poor, or charities paid the doctors.
Some hospitals and doctors charged according to income.
Provident associations were created for people on low
incomes: they paid what they could afford and donors paid

the rest. Friendly societies organised pre-payment schemes along mutual lines. Today this responsibility is assumed by government and the policy conundrum has been made more acute as a result of political involvement.

There are two further complications. First, health care may be very costly so that even a person who was self-sufficient through work in all other respects might be unable to afford it. Expenditure of this type is typically covered by insurance, allowing individuals to share in the risk of facing extraordinary costs.

Second, much ordinary medical expenditure is not extraordinary and may well be within the means of most people on ordinary incomes. However, the lower their income, the more reluctant people will be to spend on something of uncertain benefit. We often get lumps, rashes and pains or other symptoms which may soon pass or which may be the early signs of something more serious. A visit to the doctor may result in reassurance that the symptom is not significant, or that it is an early warning of a serious problem. Whether to go to see a doctor to check out something that may be trivial is a difficult judgement to make and the poorer the person the more likely they are to avoid early consultation. Historically, the difficulty was overcome by pre-payment schemes, under which small monthly payments were made to a doctor in return for regular access without fees at the time of service. For this reason, friendly societies in Britain and HMOs in America appealed to prudent people who could not afford to waste their earnings.

However, both insurance and pre-payment have disadvantages, not least that they may encourage over-use by patients. Free cover at the taxpayers' expense may have the same effect. Indeed, this is a common problem for third-party payment of all kinds. Insurers seek to overcome it by requiring co-payments or enforcing administrative rules, such as a requirement to obtain prior approval for treatment. The NHS has always relied on administrative methods such as GP gatekeepers and restricting medical resources and manpower to curtail spending.

Health Care is Different—But Not That Different

The systems in France, Germany and the UK have been based on unique approaches to the underlying characteristics of health care. France has a hybrid system which combines social insurance and a hypothecated tax. Although the amount paid by individuals is not an actuarially sound insurance premium, it reflects the price-conscious preferences of individuals for health care. Moreover, it deliberately builds in an element of co-payment to ensure that consumers are aware of the cost. For the majority of the population, not dependent on welfare benefits, it is close to a price mechanism. It also permits competition to ensure that standards are high and allows doctors outside the social insurance scheme to set market fees.

The German system also contains a price mechanism. The sickness funds are legally required to balance their books and must charge an appropriate premium. It is then applied as a percentage of each person's income. There is more of a role for GP gatekeepers in Germany than in France, but nonetheless patients enjoy freedom of choice. There is a significant amount of competition between hospitals.

Under the NHS there is an extremely weak connection between the flow of funds into the NHS and individual expectations. Whether we think in terms of wants, personal preferences or needs there is little or no link with the system of budget allocation by the Treasury. No mechanism permits our expectations to be brought into alignment with what is affordable or feasible whereas, for all the defects of the French and German systems, it is possible for individuals to make a connection between the amounts they see being deducted from their pay-slips and their experience of day-to-day access to medical services.

Neither German nor French social insurance schemes are based on actuarially sound insurance principles, but the most significant difference between them and Britain's public sector monopoly is that they have not attempted to suppress the price mechanism altogether, but rather to universalise access. In practice because social insurance works with the grain of the market it has allowed the moral purpose of universal access to be more effectively achieved. By eradicating the link between price-conscious consumers and the resources available to meet their needs the NHS has made its own moral purpose less achievable.

The Lessons

What are the lessons? The first aim of policy should be to make the market serve everyone, whether they are self-supporting through work or not. Governments should confine themselves to what they can do best and leave the rest to civil society. This implies:

1. Governments should not try to be the single payer—because rationing will be the result.

2. Nor should governments impose a single provider—because consumers cannot escape bad service and incentives to raise standards will be diminished.

3. Avoid a compulsory link with employers—because it makes it harder to move towards systems based on responsible consumers. If someone else seems to be paying, personal responsibility is diminished. However, collective purchase of insurance through *voluntary* groups (including employers) is often efficient.

4. Public policy should recognise the special nature of health care—it is partly a moral necessity and partly an ordinary consumer good. The element that is like other consumer goods is vulnerable to over-use when provided free. This recognition implies two further aims:

5. To get as close as possible to ensuring that self-sufficient people should be completely price-conscious and that dependent people should be as price-conscious as circumstances allow.

6. To ensure that people dependent on government support do not have an obviously inferior service. One approach is to make a political decision about the guaranteed standard, perhaps in the form of a 'core services' committee or an Oregon-style prioritised list. The other approach is to apply a market test which, in practice, is what countries such as France and Germany have done.

They recognise that the state cannot guarantee the standard enjoyed by the rich and so it cannot honestly promise an equal service without suppressing all private health care. But it can underwrite the standard chosen by people on middle incomes who are spending their own money. The effect of systems which combine insurance and solidarity has been to ensure that the poorest people enjoy the same level of care as the working and middle classes.

Not only have France and Germany maintained a price mechanism to permit the majority of people to influence the flow of funds into the system and avoid the widespread rationing typical of the UK, they have also encouraged competition. There is substantial private ownership of hospitals in both countries as well as a large number of independent specialists who operate from their own clinics. Consumers have real choice, whereas under the NHS, as the Government's National Plan concedes, 'the convenience of the patient can come a poor second to the convenience of the system'.

It is embarrassing for a nation to admit that it has been wrong for 50 years, but every French and German citizen has access to high-quality care—a higher standard of care than we enjoy here.

Glossary

French Chapter Abbreviations

AMG — (*Aide Médicale Générale*) Old system of medical assistance from local authorities for those on low income and unemployed. Replaced by CMU

ARH — (*Agences Régionales d'Hospitalisation*) Regional Hospital Association

CCMSA — (*Caisse Centrale de la Mutualité sociale agricole*) Agricultural workers' health insurance provider

CMU — (*Couverture Maladie Universelle*) Two-level system, introduced in January 2000, of universal health insurance based on residency, rather than employment

CNAMTS — (*Caisse Nationale d'Assurance Maladie des Travailleurs Salariés*) Health insurance for salaried workers - covers 80 per cent of the population

CPAM — (*Caisse Primaire d'Assurance Maladie*) Local social security office. Known as the '*Sécu*'

CPS — (*Carte Professionnel de Santé*) A doctor's card, required to access *carte vitale* information

CRAM — (*Caisse Régionale d'Assurance Maladie*) Regional offices, responsible for a number of CPAMs

CRDS — (*Contribution pour la Remboursement de la Dette Sociale*) A small temporary tax, introduced to help balance the social security finances

CREDES — (*Centre de recherche, d'étude et de documentation en économie de la santé*) French health economics research body

CSG — (*Contribution Sociale Généralisée*) The payroll social security contribution

CSMF — (*Confédération des Syndicats Médicaux Français*) Confédération of Medical Unions

DRASS — (*Direction Régionale des Affaires Sanitaire et Sociales*) Regional health and social affairs bureaux

DRG — Diagnosis related groups

FF — French Franc (exchange rate: £1: FF 10.4)

French Chapter Abbreviations

FMF	(*Fédération des Médecins de France*) Doctors' union representing both generalists and specialists in local, private practice
MdF	(*Médecin de Famille*) A family doctor - General Practitioner
MEDEF	The French Employers Federation
MGEN	National sickness fund for teachers
MG France	(*Médecins Généralistes de France*) GP union
MISSOC	Annual European Commission publication, summarising social protection regimes in European Union and European Economic Area member states
NHI	National Health Insurance
OECD	Organisation of Economic Cooperation and Development
ONDAM	(*Objectif National des Dépenses d'Assurance-Maladie*) Annual healthcare spending limits
RMI	(*Revenu Minimum d'Insertion*) A benefit guaranteeing those available for work, sufficient resources to live
RMO	(*Références Médicales Opposables*) Mandatory practice guidelines introduced in 1994
SAMU	(*Service d'Aide Médicale Urgente*) Specialist emergency service
SROS	(*Schéma Régionale d'Organisation Sanitaire*) General regional health services organisation plans
URCAM	(*Unions Régionales d'Assurances Maladie*) Bodies that coordinate social insurance administration at a regional level
URSSAF	(*Union pour le Recouvrement des Cotisations de Sécurité Sociale et d'Allocations familiales*) Body that collects and distributes social security contributions to the relevant organisations

French Terminology

Assurance Complémentaire	Supplementary health insurance—paid for to cover co-payments
Assurance Maladie	National Health Insurance
Avance (de frais)	Payment of costs/medical expenses at point of use
Caisses	Short form for each of the national insurance funds
Carte d'assure social	Old style medical insurance card
'Carte Vitale'	Medical/Insurance Card
Cent pour-cent	Term used when no co-payment is applied to a treatment. Equivalent of *prise en charge*
Conventionné	A doctor working within sectors 1 and 2 of the French health system
Forfait journalier	Daily, non-refundable charge in hospital
Feuille de soins	Signed statement of the treatment given and medicines prescribed—necessary for the application for refund Patients, attach vignettes to this form and return it to the CPAM so reimbursement may be processed
Loi de Financement pour la Sécurité Sociale	Annual Law of social security finance
Médecin de Famille	Family doctor - GP
Médicine libérale	The concept of unrestricted patient access to ambulatory care GPs and specialists of their choice. Also implies that physicians have freedom of prescription
Ministère de l'Emploi et de la Solidarité	The Ministry of Employment and Social Affairs—including health policy
Mutuelles	Supplementary insurers. Non-profit mutual/benefit societies

French Terminology

Non-conventionné Term to describe physicians who choose to work outside sectors 1 and 2 of the French healthcare system

Plan Juppé 1996 Reform Act

Pompiers-médicaux Semi-skilled/medically qualified firemen

Prise en charge Taken 'care of' i.e. no co-payment is required by patient

Référent Short for *Médecin Référent*. A referring GP

Tarif conventionné The tariff which *conventionné* physicians must adhere to

Tiers payant Literally meaning 'third to pay' (nearer a quarter in reality). A system whereby the patient pays only the co-payment portion up-front, rather than paying in full and being reimbursed at a later date

Ticket modérateur Element of charges health service supplied, that is not reimbursed by national insurance—the patient's contribution

Vignette In this context, a sticker, the colour of which determines what portion of pharmacy expenses will be reimbursed by the caisse

German Chapter Abbreviations

AOK	(*Allgemeine Ortskrankenkasse*) The general local insurance provider
BBV	(*Bayerische Beamten Versicherungen*) A private insurer for Beamten
BKK	(*Betriebskrankenkassen*) Company-based funds
DAK	(*Deutsche Angestellten Krankenkasse*) Insurance fund for salaried employees
DM	Deutsch Mark (exchange rate: £1: DM 3.1)
GKV	(*Gesetzliche Krankenversicherung*) Statutory Health Insurance
IKK	(*Innungskrankenkassen*) Guild insurance funds
LKK	(*Landwirtschaftliche Krankenkassen*) Agricultural workers fund
PKV	(*Privat Krankenversicherung*) Private insurance

German Terminology

Allgemeinmedizin	General medicine
Allgemeine Ortskrankenkasse	AOK Local general sickness fund
Apotheke	Pharmacy
Arzt / Ärztin	Doctor (m/f)
Arzt für allgemeine	General Practitioner
Augenarzt	Eye specialist
Beamte / in	Permanent civil servant (m/f)
Beihilfe	Aid, assistance, allowance (eg for Beamte)
Betriebskrankenkasse, BKK	Company sickness fund
Bundesarztekammer	German Medical Association
Bundesministerium für Gesundheit	Federal Health Ministry
Chip-karte	Smart card proving membership of an insurance fund
Ersatzkasse	Substitute health insurance funds
Frauenarzt	Specialist gynaecologist
Hausarzt / ärztin	GP (m/f)
Innungskrankenkasse, IKK	Guild health insurance fund
Internist	Internal specialist doctor
Kassenarztliche Bundesvereiningung (KBV)	Federal Association of Sickness Fund Doctors
Kinderspezialist	Specialist children's physician

German Terminology

Kostenübernamhe	Undertaking to pay costs (of health care)
Kostenübernahmerschein	Form from the insurance company stating that it (the company) will pay for treatment costs in general nursing care
Krankenkasse / n	Sickness fund/s
Krankenschein	Insurance certificate, now supplanted by Chip-karten
Krankenversicherung	Sickness insurance
Notwendigkeitsbesheiningung	Certificate stating the patient's need for hospital treatment
Pfelgeversicherung	(Long-term) care insurance
Seehofer Reform Act	The Seehofer Reform of 1992 (In force 1993)
Sozialamt	Social Welfare Office
Sozialhilfe	Social Welfare (benefits)
Techniker Krankenkasse	One of the larger GKV insurers
Überweisung	Referral
Überweisungsschein	Referral note - from a doctor

Notes

1. French and Germany: The Consumer's View

1   Mossialos, E., 'Citizen's views on health systems in the 15 member states of the European Union', *Health Economics*, Vol. 6, pp. 109-16, and Eurobarometer survey. 1997.

2   Jabubowski, E., *Health Care Systems in the EU: A Comparative Study*, E. P. Working Paper, SACO 101/rev. EN, European Parliament, 1998.

3   World Health Organisation, *'World Health Report 2000'*, Geneva, WHO, 2000. The criteria according to which the conclusions of the WHO 2000 Report were reached have been subject to criticism from a wide range of sources.

4   The interviews reported were not randomly selected. They were chosen from among the people we spoke to because they added insights which a bare-bones technical description of a health system cannot provide. To ensure that broad comparisons could be made between French, German and British healthcare systems, the interviews were semi-structured, with questions relating to funding, ambulatory and secondary provision, and recent healthcare reforms.

5   Employers pay 12.8 per cent of an employee's salary. See p. 32 for more contribution details.

6   Supplementary insurance paid for by 80 per cent of the French, to cover co-payments—the portion of fees not reimbursed by the sickness funds following payment at point of use—*'avance de frais'*. This user payment is a key element of the French healthcare system. See 'CMU' for recent changes affecting those who could not afford to pay for this extra insurance.

7   The monetary conversion rates used in this were fixed on 31 August 2001: £1=FF 10.4; £1=DM 3.1.

8   Privacy is routine in private hospitals. Public hospitals may also have single-bedded rooms, but 2-4 beds per room would be more common.

9   FF 150 being the standard *conventionné*—that is sector 1—specialist's fee.

10 By contrast, *mutuelles* usually reimburse more quickly —as failure to do so may cause a member to transfer to a competitor.

11 When the French refer to a *médecin de famille*, they imply a degree of fidelity to one GP—usually while children and/or elderly relatives are dependent.

12 This means that treatment is *prise en charge* —provided for free, without a *ticket modérateur*.

13 UK doctors have a financial incentive to prescribe the 'pill', as do French doctors, but in France provision is made for a number of paid consultations.

14 *Techniker* is one of the larger *Krankenkassen*—health insurance providers. See pp. 55-58 for further details about German health insurers.

15 *Allgemeine Ortskrankenkasse* (AOK): the largest German health insurance organisation—covering about 40 per cent of the insured.

16 *Deutsche Angestellten Krankenkasse* (DAK)—prior to 1996 membership was compulsory for certain salaried employees.

17 Sickness fund membership was liberalised following the second stage of reforms which were introduced by the 1993 Healthcare Structural Reform Act—the 'Seehofer Reform'. Patients base their choice between funds on a number of factors including the benefits included, above and beyond those detailed in the *Sozialgestetzbuch Fünftes Buch* (SGB V), *Gesetzliche Krankenversicherung*, 2000, (as amended by the *GKV-Gesundheitsreform 2000*) which all insurers must offer.

18 GPs or family doctors are called *Hausarzt / ärztin* (masc/fem).

19 Children in Germany attend specialist facilities throughout their youth—with specially tailored equipment. 'Paediatrician' does not have the same meaning as in the UK. When attending the child-doctor, she would take along the medical prevention 'exercise book', given to all German children.

20   The co-payment for the smallest prescription
      package.

21   See p. 62 for details.

22   The DM 1000 (c£330) figure is not standard across
      the Federal Republic—it might vary according to the
      insurer and type of policy purchased, also according
      to the agreements that healthcare providers have
      made with insurers.

23   The existence or threat of rationing in Germany is
      the subject of some debate. For example see
      Redwood H., *Why Ration Health Care?*, London:
      Civitas, 2000.

24   'Dual system'—whereby most are GKV insured while
      some are wholly privately (PKV) insured and might
      therefore receive an arguably higher standard of
      treatment—in terms of speed of obtaining an
      appointment, length of that appointment, waiting
      time before treatment, privacy, and so forth. This
      contrast is particularly stark when comparing the
      standard of service received by some AOK members,
      with that of the privately insured. Among our
      interviewees, with the exception of one content AOK
      member, AOK was thought of as the 'insurer of last
      resort'—one to avoid if at all possible. Some suggest
      that reference to a 'dual system' is inaccurate, as
      there are three, four, or more levels of service.

25   This compulsory pension insurance is called
      Retensversicherung.

26   German pensions are about 70 per cent of final
      salary.

27   The proceeding two paragraphs are based on
      information from the publications: Kappler, A. and
      Reichart, S. (eds.), *Facts about Germany,* Press and
      Information Office of the Federal Government 1999;
      The Federal Ministry of Labour and Social Affairs,
      Social Security at a Glance, 1999; Graig, L., *Health
      of Nations: An International Perspective on US
      Health Care Reform,* 3rd edn, Washington DC:
      Congressional Quarterly Inc., 1999; European
      Commission, DG V, *Your Social Security Rights
      When Moving Within the European Union,*
      Luxembourg: Office for Official Publications of the

European Communities, 1995; and European Commission, *MISSOC 2000, Social Protection in the EU Member States and the European Economic Area*, Luxembourg: Office for Official Publications of the European Communities, 2001.

28 See p. 64 for more details.

29 Herr Braun's figures.

30 Details of transport entitlements are found in Chapter 3 of the *Sozialgesetzbuch*, V. This applies to GKV and PKV members, though the level of benefits in kind might vary considerably among the privately insured.

2: France: The System

1 Bouckaert G. and Pollitt C., *Comparative Public Management in OECD Countries*, Oxford University Press, 1999.

2 CIA, *The World Factbook - France*, 2000. www.odci.gov/cia/publications/factbook

3 Lacronique, J-F., 'Health Services in France', in Raffel, M. (ed.), *Comparative Health Systems*, 2nd edn, Penn State: Pennsylvania State University Press, 1984.

4 Capul, J-Y., *Emploi et Protection Sociale*, No. 202, Cahiers Francais, July-September 1999.

5 Capul, *Emploi et Protection Sociale*, 1999.

6 There was a modest deficit in 2000. Imai, Y., Jacobzone, S. and Lenain, P., in 'The Changing Health System in France' (Economics Department Working Paper 269, ECO/WKP(2000)42, OECD, 2000), consider that a permanent solution to the funding crisis has not yet been found.

7 Sorau, A., Bary, I. and Couvelaere, J., *The French Healthcare Sector*, Paris: British Embassy, March 2000.

8 Material from Freeman, R., *The Politics of Health in Europe*, European Policy Research Unit Series, Manchester University Press, 2000; Capul, *Emploi et Protection Sociale*, 1999; Lacronique, 'Health Services in France', 1984.

9   Jabubowski, E., *Health Care Systems in the EU: a Comparative Study*, European Parliament Working Paper, SACO 101/rev. EN, 1998.

10   Freeman, *The Politics of Health in Europe*, 2000.

11   Imai, Jacobzone, and Lenain, 'The Changing Health System in France', 2000.

12   Capul, *Emploi et Protection Sociale*, 1999.

13   Duriez, M., *Le Système de Santé en France*, Paris: Haut Comite de Santé Publique, 2000. www.sante.gouv.fr/htm/minister/systsan.htm

14   Sources: Freeman, *The Politics of Health in Europe*, 2000; Godt, P., (1996), 'The politics of health care reform in France', paper presented to workshop, 'Beyond the Health Care State. New Dimensions in Health Politics in Europe', ECPR Joint Sessions of Workshops, Oslo, 29 March-3 April. Cited in Freeman, *The Politics of Health in Europe*, 2000. Also see Pomey, M.-P. and Poullier, J.P., 'France's Health Policy Conundrum', in Raffel, *Health Care and Reform in Industrialised Countries*, 1997.

15   Jabubowski, *Health Care Systems in the EU: a Comparative Study*, 1998; and Pomey and Poullier, 'France's Health Policy Conundrum', 1997.

16   Duriez, *Le Système de Santé en France*, 2000.

17   Palier, B., 'A "Liberal" Dynamic in the Transformation of the French Social Welfare System', in Clasen, J. (ed.), *Social Insurance in Europe*, Bristol: Policy Press, 1997. Cited in Freeman, *The Politics of Health in Europe*, 2000.

18   Duriez, *Le Système de Santé en France*, 2000.

19   Freeman, *The Politics of Health in Europe*, 2000.

20   A temporary social debt tax—*cotisation pour le remboursement de la dette sociale* (CRDS)—has also been introduced.

21   Redwood, H., *Why Ration Health Care?*, London: Civitas, 2000.

22 Bocognano, A., Couffinhal, A., Dumesnil, S. and Grignon, M., *La Complémentaire maladie en France: qui bénéfice de quels remboursements*, Biblio No. 1317, CREDES, Paris, 2000. See CMU on p. 38.

23 Lacronique, 'Health Services in France', 1984.

24 For example, this rationale behind co-payments is mentioned by Duriez, M., Lancry, P-J., Lequet-Slama, D. and Sandier, S., *'Le Système de Santé en France'*, Que sais-je?, No. 3066, Presses Universitaires de France, 1996.

25 European Commission, *MISSOC, 2000, Social Protection in the EU Member States and the European Economic Area*, 2001. http://vosdroits.service-public.fr
  Co-payment for hospital treatment does not apply to surgery, nor for treatment above a certain level on the official scale of sicknesses, nor for treatment after the 31st day of hospitalisation. The category 'Irreplaceable (vital) or costly' is translated from 'les medicaments irremplacables ou couteux pour les affections graves et invalidantes', in Duriez, Lancry *et al*, *Le Système de Santé en France*, 1996.

26 Dourgnon, P. and Grignon, M., *Le tiers-payant est-il inflationniste?* No 1296 CREDES, Paris, 2000.

27 Otherwise known as *'éxoneration du ticket modérateur'*.

28 Translated from Duriez, Lancry *et al*, *Le Système de Santé en France*, 1996.

29 Claims are made whenever medical expenses are incurred. CNAMTS reimbursement statements are received roughly monthly.

30 La Premiere Ministre, (Lionel, Jospin), *L'égal accès de tous a la santé*, La Lettre du Gouvernement, No. 60, Service d'information du Gouvernement, February 1999.

31 See Boisguérin, B., *Les bénéficaires de la couverture maladie universelle au 30 septembre 2000*, No. 96, DREES, Études et Résultats, Ministère de l'Emploi et de la solidarité, 2000. Those without medical cover included the homeless, illegal immigrants, and some of the very wealthy.

32   Jabubowski, *Health Care Systems in the EU: a Comparative Study*, 1998.

33   FF 5400 for two people, FF 6480 for three, FF 7560 for four people and FF 1440 for each additional person thereafter. Figures taken from: http://vosdroits.service-publique.fr

34   *'Revenue minimum d'insertion'*—a social security benefit available to all those available for work, over the age of 25, RMI guarantees sufficient resources to live.

35   Boisguérin, *Les bénéficaires de la couverture maladie universelle au 30 septembre 2000*, 2000.

36   Imai, Jacobzone, and Lenain, 'The Changing Health System in France', 2000; and Boisguérin, *Les bénéficaires de la couverture maladie universelle au 30 septembre 2000*, 2000.

37   Bernard Brunhes Consultants, *Universal Health Cover, (Couverture Maladie Universelle, CMU)*, 2000; Ministère de l'Emploi et de la solidarité and Les Caisses D'Assurance Maladie, *La Couverture Maladie Universelle*, Information leaflet, 2000; Bocogano, A., Couffinhal, A., Dumesnil, S. and Grignon, M., *La Complémentaire maladie en France: qui bénéfice de quels remboursements*. Questions d'économie de la santé, No. 32, CREDES, Paris, October 2000; Imai, Jacobzone, and Lenain, 'The Changing Health System in France', 2000; and Boisguérin, *Les bénéficaires de la couverture maladie universelle au 30 septembre 2000*, 2000.

38   Entry to practice under health insurance is open to all doctors who qualified in France. Professional Licensing is managed by the *Ordre des Medecins,* established in 1940, is organised at departmental, regional and national levels. In the early 1970s a *numerus clausus* was introduced in French medical schools—the aim being to reduce what was an excessive number of medical practitioners. For similar reasons, on some occasions, access to sector-2 has been subject to restriction. Shortages of doctors in certain hospital roles led to the introduction of a mandatory hospital internship for medical students. Unlike France, in Germany, there is no *numerus*

clausus for medical students because the German constitution guarantees the right to medical education subject only to entry qualifications. Instead, since the Health Care Reform Act 1992, the Regional Physicians' Associations have geographically and by specialism restricted the settlement of new doctors. In 1995 there was no state where all sub-regions were open for all specialties, however, there were openings for all specialties elsewhere in the federal republic. As of 1999 the number of doctors has been limited to the actual requirements basis of legally fixed ratios. At the same time, an age limit of 68 years was introduced. (See Busse, R., *Health Care Systems in Transition: Germany*, European Observatory on Health Care Systems, 2000; and Graig, *Health of Nations*, 1999, for details).

39 Ministry of Employment and Solidarity, *Health in France 1994-1998*, Ministry of Employment and Solidarity High Committee on Public Health, Paris, 1998. Physicians are over-represented in major metropolitan areas and throughout the south of France, while many other rural areas, particularly in the north, have much lower physician density per 1,000.

40 Duriez, *Le Système de Santé en France*, 2000.

41 Poullier, J-P. and Sandier, S., 'France', in *Journal of Health Politics, Policy and Law*, Vol. 25, No. 5, October 2000.

42 Poullier and Sandier, 'France', 2000.

43 The number 175,000 includes physicians working in both primary and secondary care. Duriez, *Le Système de Santé en France*, 2000.

44 Jabubowski, *Health Care Systems in the EU: a Comparative Study*, 1998.

45 Psychiatrists charge FF 225 (about £22).

46 Dorozynski uses the latter expression in Dorozynski A., 'France launches plan to control health costs', in *British Medical Journal*, 1998; 317:164.

47   Lancry, P.-J., and Sandier, S., 'Twenty years of cures
      for the French health care system', in Mossialos, E.
      and Le Grand, J. (eds.), *Health Care and Cost
      Containment in the EU*, Ashgate, 1999.

48   Aguzzoli, A., Alignon, A., Com-Ruelle, L. and Frérot,
      L., *Choisir d'avoir un médicin référent*, Biblio, No.
      1281, CREDES, Paris,1999.

49   Imai, Jacobzone, and Lenain, 'The Changing Health
      System in France', 2000.

50   Jabubowski, *Health Care Systems in the EU: a
      Comparative Study*, 1998;
      also see www.finances.gouv.fr

51   Freeman, *The Politics of Health in Europe*, 2000.

52   Figures and definitions are compiled from
      www.sante.gouv.fr; Duriez, *Le Système de Santé en
      France*, 2000; Duriez, Lancry *et al*, *Le Système de
      Santé en France*, 1996; Lacronique, 'Health Services
      in France', 1984.

53   Jabubowski, *Health Care Systems in the EU: a
      Comparative Study*, 1998.

54   Jabubowski, *Health Care Systems in the EU: a
      Comparative Study*, 1998.

55   Lancry and Sandier, 'Twenty years of cures for the
      French health care system', 1999.

56   Jabubowski, *Health Care Systems in the EU: a
      Comparative Study*, 1998.

57   Freeman, *The Politics of Health in Europe*, 2000.

58   Freeman, *The Politics of Health in Europe*, 2000.

59   Reimbursement of 35 per cent is made for
      *'médicaments de confort'—pour le traitement
      symptomatique d'affection sans caractère de gravité*.
      Translated from Duriez, Lancry *et al*, *Le Système de
      Santé en France*, 1996, as 'drugs mainly meant for
      troubles or affections normally without gravity'. I.e.
      'non-essential drugs', or those for 'non-serious
      diseases' such as medicines for pain relief.
      Reimbursement of 65 per cent is made for *'des
      médicaments s'adressant à des pathologies graves'*.
      Translated from Duriez, Lancry *et al*, *Le Système de*

Santé en France, 1996, as the majority of 'necessary' drugs.

While full reimbursement is made for *'les médicaments irremplacables ou couteux pour les affections graves et invalidantes'*. Translated from Duriez, Lancry *et al, Le Système de Santé en France*, Que sais-je?, 1996, as drugs for irreplaceable or costly conditions of serious or debilitating nature.

60   From Redwood, *Why Ration Health Care?*, 2000.

61   Capul, *Emploi et Protection Sociale*, 1999.

62   Capul, *Emploi et Protection Sociale*, 1999.

63   CREDES: Centre de Recherche D'Étude et de Documentation en Économie de la Santé. 'Centre for Research and Documentation in Health Economics'.

64   This *CREDES* report is cited by Redwood, *Why Ration Health Care?*, 2000.

65   Freeman, *The Politics of Health in Europe*, 2000.

66   Note, this figure of 60 per cent relates to primary care benefits, and pharmaceutical expenditure. The level of public finance is much higher in the hospital sector, and much lower for dental benefits. See Lancry and Sandier, 'Twenty years of cures for the French health care system', 1999.

67   Capul, *Emploi et Protection Sociale*, 1999.

68   Freeman, *The Politics of Health in Europe*, 2000.

69   Duran-Zaleski, I., Colin, C. and Blum-Boisgard, C., 'An attempt to save money by using mandatory practice guidelines in France', in *British Medical Journal*, 1997; 315 (7113):943.

70   Dorozyski, A, 'French doctors agitated over cash "bonus"', in *British Medical Journal*, 2000; 321:528.

71   Dorozyski, 'French doctors agitated over cash "bonus"', 2000.

3: Germany: the System

1   CIA, *The World Factbook - Germany*, 2000.
www.odci.gov/cia/publications/factbook

2   For example, see the following: Ulrich, V., 'Health
     Care in Germany: Structure, Expenditure and
     Prospects', in McArthur, W., Ramsay, C. and
     Walker, M. (eds.), *Healthy Incentives: Canadian
     Health Reform in an International Context*, The
     Fraser Institute, 1996; Henke, K.-D., Ade, C. and
     Murray, M., 'The German health care system:
     structures and changes', in *Journal of Clinical
     Anesthesia*, 6, 1994, pp. 252-62. Cited by Ulrich,
     'Health Care in Germany: Structure, Expenditure
     and Prospects', 1996; Webber, D., 'Health Policy and
     the Christian-Liberal Coalition in West Germany:
     the Conflicts over the Health Insurance Reform
     1987-8', in Altenstetter, C. and Haywood, S. (eds.),
     Comparative Health Policy and the New Right, St
     Martins, 1991; Altenstetter, C., 'An end to a
     consensus on health care in the Federal Republic of
     Germany?', *Journal of Health Politics, Policy and
     Law*, 12, 1987, pp. 505-36.

3   Webber, 'Health insurance reform in the Federal
     Republic of Germany', 1991. Also see Altenstetter,
     C., 'From Solidarity to Market Competition? Values
     Structure, and Strategy in German Health Policy,
     1883-1997', in Powell, F. and Wessen, A. (eds.),
     Health Care Systems in Transition, Sage
     Publications, 1999.
         The management of the 13 *Ersatzkassen* differs,
     with only representatives of the insured sitting on
     an elected assembly—see Busse, R., *Health Care
     Systems in Transition: Germany*, European
     Observatory on Health Care Systems, 2000.

4   Altenstetter, C., (1987), 'An end to a consensus on
     health care in the Federal Republic of Germany?
     Journal of Health Politics, Policy and Law, 12, 1987,
     pp. 505-36; Altenstetter, C., *Krankenhausbedarf-
     splannung: Was brachte sie wirklich?*, Munich:
     Oldenbourg, 1985. Cited by Altenstetter, 'From
     Solidarity to Market Competition? Values Structure,
     and Strategy in German Health Policy, 1883-1997',
     1999.

5   Behagel, K., *Kostendämpfung und ärztliche
     Interssenvertretung: Ein Verbandssytem unter Streß*.
     Frankfurt: Campus, 1994. Cited by Altenstetter,
     'From Solidarity to Market Competition? Values

Structure, and Strategy in German Health Policy, 1883-1997', 1999.

6   Bundesministerium für Gesundheit (Federal Ministry of Health), *Health Care in Germany*, Federal Ministry of Health, Meid + Partner, Bonn, 1997.

7   Bundesministerium für Gesundheit, *Health Care in Germany*, 1997; Bundesministerium für Gesundheit, Inter Nationes, *Health Care in Germany*, Basis-info 12-1997, In-Press, 1997; Bundesministerium für Gesundheit, *Terms of Reference*, December 1998; and Health Ministry, *Health Care in Germany*, website - 2001, www.bmgesundheit.de/eng/health

8   Jabubowski, E., *Health Care Systems in the EU: a Comparative Study*, European Parliament Working Paper, SACO 101/rev. EN, European Parliament, 1998.

9   Hoffmeyer, U., 'The Health Care System in Germany' in Hoffmeyer, U.K. and McCarthy, T. R. (eds.), *Financing Health Care*, Vol. 1, Dortrecht, the Netherlands: Kluwer Academic Publishers, 1994, pp. 419-512. Cited by Altenstetter, 'From Solidarity to Market Competition? Values Structure, and Strategy in German Health Policy, 1883-1997', 1999.

10   The threshold is DM 6525 per month, (about £2,100) in 2001. Of the 21 per cent of the population whose income is above this threshold, more than two-thirds chose to remain GKV insured. Thomson and Mossialos put the figure at 23 per cent of those with the option. [Thomson, S. and Mossialos, E., 'The demand for private health insurance in Germany', in *Euro Observer*, No. 4, Vol. 12, 2001.]

11   This material is compiled from European Commission, *MISSOC 2000, Social Protection in EU Member States and the European Economic Area*, 2001; European Commission, *Your Social Security Rights When Moving within the European Union* 1995; and Iglehart, J., 'Health policy report: Germany's health care system', *New England Journal of Medicine*, Vol. 324, 1991, pp. 503-08.

12   There is an annual contributions ceiling. Thus some of the very well off while paying more in absolute terms pay less proportionately than the less-well-off. I.e. the system is mildly regressive.

13   European Commission, *Your Social Security Rights When Moving within the European Union,* 1995; and Federal Ministry of Labour and Social affairs, *Social Security at a Glance,* Federal Ministry of Labour and Social affairs, 1999.

14   Bundesministerium für Gesundheit, *Health Care in Germany,* Meid + Partner, Bonn, 1997.

15   Note, this refers to GKV insurance members only; the privately insured generally pay for ambulatory care (by invoice) and are subsequently by their insurer.

16   Graig, L., *Health of Nations: An International Perspective on US Health Care Reform,* 3rd edn, Washington DC: Congressional Quarterly Inc., 1999.

17   Kappler, A. and Reichart, S. (eds.), *Facts about Germany,* Press and Information Office of the Federal Government 1999.

18   Graig, *Health of Nations,* 1999; Busse, *Health Care Systems in Transition: Germany,* 2000; European Commission, *MISSOC, 2000, Social Protection in EU Member States and the European Economic Area,* 2001; Comité Européen des Assurances, *Health Insurance in Europe,* CEA, Paris, 1997.

19   Abel-Smith, B. and Mossialos, E., 'Cost containment and health care reform: a study of the European Union health policy', *Health Policy,* 28, 1994, pp. 89-132.
      A number of company-based BKK funds still operate a closed membership system, but it is estimated that over 80 per cent of enrolees are free to choose their insurer (Oliver, A., in *Risk Adjusting Health Care Resource Allocations: Theory and practice in the United Kingdom, the Netherlands and Germany,* London: Office of Health Economics, 1999).

20   Bundesministerium für Gesundheit, *Health Care in Germany*, Meid + Partner, Bonn, 1997. Note, that it is said that some employers push workers to enrol with the fund with the lowest contribution rates by paying the minimum contribution if they chose a more expensive fund.

21   Scheil-Adlung, X., 'Steering the healthcare ship: effects of market incentives to control costs in selected OECD countries', *International Social Security Review*, 5, No. 1, 1998. Cited by Graig, *Health of Nations*, 1999; on competition also see Ulrich, 'Health Care in Germany: Structure, Expenditure and Prospects', 1996; and Brown, L.D. and Amelung V.E., 'Manacled competition: market reforms in German health care', *Health Affairs*, Vol. 18, No. 3, 1999.

22   List compiled from the following sources: European Commission, 1995; Busse, *Health Care Systems in Transition: Germany*, 2000; Graig, *Health of Nations,* 1999; Allgemeine Ortskrankenkasse, *Social Security with the AOK,*, Praxis, Aktuell 2000; Allgemeine Ortskrankenkasse, Studies, Studiothek, AOK, 1999.

23   Bundesministerium für Gesundheit, website - 2001, www.bmgesundheit.de/eng/health

24   See Brown, and Amelung, 'Manacled competition', 1999. Also see Busse, *Health Care Systems in Transition: Germany*, 2000.

25   Graig, *Health of Nations*, 1999.

26   Figures from Busse, *Health Care Systems in Transition: Germany*, 2000.

27   Compiled from Graig, *Health of Nations*, 1999; Busse, *Health Care Systems in Transition: Germany*, 2000; and Freeman, *The Politics of Health in Europe*, 2000.

28   For more detailed discussion of this and other risk equalisation schemes see Oliver, *Risk Adjusting Health Care Resource Allocation*, 1999. Also see, Rice, N. and Smith, P., *Approaches to Capitation and Risk Adjustment in Health Care: An International Survey*, The University of York, CHE, 1999.

29   Graig, *Health of Nations*, 1999.

30   Altenstetter, 'From Solidarity to Market Competition?', 1999.

31   Altenstetter, 'From Solidarity to Market Competition?', 1999.

32   See Oliver, *Risk Adjusting Health Care Resource Allocation*, 1999. Also see Altenstetter, 'From Solidarity to Market Competition?', 1999.

33   See Busse, *Health Care Systems in Transition: Germany*, 2000; and Brown, and Amelung, 'Manacled competition', 1999.

34   Federal Health Ministry, *Health Care in Germany*, website - 2001; www.bvmed.de/text/reimbursement.htm -

35   Federal Health Ministry, *Health Care in Germany*, website - 2001.

36   Federal Health Ministry, *Health Care in Germany*, website - 2001; and European Commission, *MISSOC 2000, Social Protection in EU Member States and the European Economic Area*, 2001.

37   Altenstetter, 'From Solidarity to Market Competition?', 1999.

38   Bundesministerium für Gesundheit, *Health Care in Germany*, Meid + Partner, Bonn, 1997.

39   List compiled from: Bundesministerium für Gesundheit, *Health Care in Germany*, Meid + Partner, Bonn, 1997; Federal Health Ministry, *Health Care in Germany*, website - 2001; and Busse, *Health Care Systems in Transition: Germany*, 2000.

40   Altenstetter, 'From solidarity to market competition? Values structure, and strategy in German health policy, 1883-1997', 1999.

41   List compiled from: European Commission, *MISSOC 2000, Social Protection in EU Member States and the European Economic Area*, 2001; European Commission, *Your Social Security Rights When Moving within the European Union* 1995; Ulrich, 'Health Care in Germany: Structure, Expenditure and

Prospects', 1996; Brown, and Amelung, 'Manacled competition',1999.

42 Federal Ministry of Labour and Social affairs, *Social Security at a Glance*. Federal Ministry of Labour and Social affairs, 1999.

43 Busse, R. and Howorth, C., 'Cost containment in Germany: twenty years experience', in Mossialos, E. and Le Grand, J. (eds), *Health Care and Cost Containment in the European Union*, Ashgate Publishing Limited, 1999.

44 Sources: Direction des communications ministère de la Santé et des Services sociaux du Québec., DIRIS, Ministère de l'Emploi et de la Solidarité, and SESI, '*Health Indicators. International Comparisons. 15 years of evolution*, 1998 (English) edn, Direction des communications ministère de la Santé et des Services sociaux du Québec, 1998; Brown, and Amelung, 'Manacled competition', 1999; Federal Ministry of Labour and Social affairs, *Social Security at a Glance*, 1999.

45 Kelly-Gagnon, M., *Universal Care and Freedom of Choice are Not Mutually Exclusive*, IEDM Healthcare Solutions. www.iedm.org/chronique/may-00.en

46 Sources: Graig, *Health of Nations*, 1999; Comité Européen des Assurances, *Health Insurance in Europe, 1997*, CEA Papers, 1997.

47 Sources: Comité Européen des Assurances, Private Health Insurance in Europe, CEA Papers, Nr 2, Paris, May 1983; Ulrich, 'Health Care in Germany: Structure, Expenditure and Prospects', 1996; and Verband der Privaten Krankenversicherung e.V. (Association of Private Health Insurers) *Private Health Insurance, Facts and Figures 1999/2000*, Cologne, October 2000.

48 Graig, *Health of Nations*, 1999; Thomson and Mossialos, 'The demand for private health insurance in Germany', 2001.

49 Sources: Bundesministerium für Gesundheit, *Health Care in Germany*, Meid + Partner, Bonn, 1997; Graig, *Health of Nations*, 1999; Comité Européen des

Assurances *Health Insurance in Europe*, 1997; and, Verband der Privaten Krankenversicherung e.V. (Association of Private Health Insurers) *Private Health Insurance, Facts and Figures 1999/2000*, 2000.

50   Sources: see note 68.

51   However, employers will only pay up to half the average contribution that would go to a GKV fund member.

52   Graig, *Health of Nations*, 1999.

53   Verband der Privaten Krankenversicherung e.V. *Private Health Insurance, Facts and Figures 1999/2000*, 2000.

54   Sources: Comité Européen des Assurances, *Health Insurance in Europe*, 1997; and Verband der Privaten Krankenversicherung e.V, *Private Health Insurance, Facts and Figures 1999/2000*, 2000.

55   Graig, *Health of Nations*, 1999.

56   Busse, *Health Care Systems in Transition: Germany*, 2000.

57   Mullen, F., 'The "Mona Lisa" of Health Policy: Primary Care at Home and Abroad', *Health Affairs*, 17, No. 2, 1998. Cited in Graig *Health of Nations*, 1999.

58   Figures in this section are from the OECD, *Health Data 2001*, CD-Rom, 2001.

59   Graig, *Health of Nations*, 1999.

60   Busse, *Health Care Systems in Transition. Germany*, 2000.

61   Statistiches Bundesamt, *Health Report for Germany, Abridged Version*. 'Health Monitoring of the Federation', Federal Statistics Office, 1998.

62   Busse, *Health Care Systems in Transition: Germany*, 2000.

63   Graig, *Health of Nations*, 1999.

64   There are 36 recognised medical specialities and 50 sub-specialities (Busse, 2000).

65 Busse, and Howorth, 'Cost containment in Germany: twenty years experience', 1999.

66 Bundesministerium für Gesundheit, *Health Care in Germany*, Meid + Partner, Bonn, 1997.

67 US Department of State, *Electro-Medical Equipment*, Industrial Sector Analysis, 1999.

68 Sources: Busse, *Health Care Systems in Transition. Germany*, 2000; Graig, *Health of Nations*, 1999; and Statisches Bundesamt, *Health Report for Germany, Abridged Version*, 1998.

69 Ulrich, 'Health Care in Germany: Structure, Expenditure and Prospects', 1996; Busse, *Health Care Systems in Transition: Germany*, 2000.

70 Kirkman-Liff, B., 'Health care cost containment in Germany', in Powell and Wessen (eds.), *Health Care Systems in Transition*, 1999.

71 Kirkman-Liff, 'Health care cost containment in Germany', 1999.

72 Kirkman-Liff, 'Health care cost containment in Germany', 1999.

73 See Busse, *Health Care Systems in Transition: Germany*, 2000. Also see Ulrich, Ulrich, 'Health Care in Germany: Structure, Expenditure and Prospects', 1996; and Kirkman-Liff, 'Health care cost containment in Germany', 1999.

74 Abel-Smith, and Mossialos, 'Cost containment and health care reform: a study of the European Union health policy', 1994 ; and World Health Organisation (WHO), *Highlights on Health in Germany, 1997*, Copenhagen, 1999.

75 Figures are from OECD *Health Data 2001*, CD-Rom, Paris, OECD and CREDES, 2001.

76 World Health Organisation, *Highlights on Health in Germany, 1997*, 1999.

77 europa.eu.int/scadplus/citizens/en/de/1084.htm

78 Ulrich, 'Health Care in Germany: Structure, Expenditure and Prospects', 1996.

79   Ulrich, 'Health Care in Germany: Structure, Expenditure and Prospects', 1996; Graig, *Health of Nations*, 1999; and Busse, *Health Care Systems in Transition: Germany*, 2000.

80   www.bvmed.de/text/reimbursement.htm - Reimbursement and pricing of medical devices in Germany. 2000; Busse, R.,'Germany opts for Australian Diagnosis-Related Groups', *Euro Observer*, Vol. 2, No. 3, European Observatory on Health Care Systems, 2000.

81   Graig, *Health of Nations*, 1999.

82   Federal Health Ministry—*'Terms of Reference'*, December 1998.

83   Pflege, Band 10, 1997, Heft 2, Seiten 102-112. Verlag hans Huber, Bern.

84   Sources: Embassy of the Federal Republic of Germany, 'Labour and Social Affairs, Health I: The cost of health: 14.3 per cent of GDP', and 'Labour and Social Affairs, Health II: Care insurance: an anniversary and a goal', Press Release, Embassy of the Federal Republic of Germany, No 4/2000; Bundesministerium für Gesundheit, *Health Care in Germany*, Meid + Partner, Bonn, 1997; and Federal Health Ministry, *Health Care in Germany*, website - 2001.

85   Federal Health Ministry, *Health Care in Germany*, website - 2001.

86   Embassy of the Federal Republic of Germany, Labour and Social Affairs, 'Health I: The cost of health: 14.3 per cent of GDP'; and 'Health II: Care insurance: an anniversary and a goal', Press Release, Embassy of the Federal Republic of Germany, No 4/2000.

87   Kappler, A. and Reichart, S. (eds.), *Facts About Germany*, Press and Information Office of the Federal Government, 1999.

88   Statistiches Bundesamt, *Health Report for Germany, Abridged Version*, 1998; and US International Trade Commission, *Pricing of Prescription Drugs*, Publication 3333, US ITC, 2000.

89   Busse, *Health Care Systems in Transition: Germany*, 2000; and US ITC, *Pricing of Prescription Drugs*, 2000.

90   Tuffs, A., 'German doctors are unhappy about drugs budget', in *British Medical Journal*, 1999;319:536; and US ITC, *Pricing of Prescription Drugs*, 2000.

91   Ulrich, 'Health Care in Germany: Structure, Expenditure and Prospects', 1996; Jabubowski, *Health Care Systems in the EU: a Comparative Study*, 1998.

92   Busse, *Health Care Systems in Transition: Germany*, 2000; and US ITC, *Pricing of Prescription Drugs*, 2000.

93   Kappler and Reichart (eds.), *Facts about Germany*, 1999.

94   Redwood, *Why Ration Health Care?*, 2000.

95   Numerous such examples were cited in November 1999 in an article entitled 'Teure Patienten unerwunscht' ('Expensive Patients unwelcome') in *Die Zeit*.

96   Powell and Wessen (eds.), *Health Care Systems in Transition*, 1999.

97   US ITC, *Pricing of Prescription Drugs*, 2000. Our interviewees confirmed this differential access to innovative treatments between the privately and statutorily insured.

98   US ITC, *Pricing of Prescription Drugs*, 2000, appendix 2, p. 23.

99   Graig, *Health of Nations*, 1999.

100   Redwood, *Why Ration Health Care?*, 2000.

101   Ulrich, 'Health Care in Germany: Structure, Expenditure and Prospects', 1996.

102   Ulrich, 'Health Care in Germany: Structure, Expenditure and Prospects', 1996.

103   For more details of the contents of each of these reform acts, see Graig, *Health of Nations*, 1999; Powell and Wessen (eds.), *Health Care Systems in Transition*, 1999; Freeman, *The Politics of Health in*

Europe, 2000; Mossialos and Le Grand, J. (eds), *Health Care and Cost Containment in the European Union*, 1999; Busse, *Health Care Systems in Transition: Germany*, 2000; and the Federal Health Ministry, *Health Care in Germany*, website - 2001.

104   Graig, *Health of Nations*, 1999.

105   Direction des communications ministère de la Santé et des Services sociaux du Québec, DIRIS, Ministère de l'Emploi et de la Solidarité, and SESI, *Health Indicators. International Comparisons: 15 Years of Evolution*, 1998; Graig, *Health of Nations*, 1999; and Busse, *Health Care Systems in Transition: Germany*, 2000.

106   Graig, *Health of Nations*, 1999.

107   Quoted by Altenstetter, 'From solidarity to market competition? Values structure, and strategy in German health policy, 1883-1997', 1999.

108   Graig, *Health of Nations*, 1999.

109   Freeman, *The Politics of Health in Europe*, 2000; Busse, *Health Care Systems in Transition: Germany*, 2000.

110   Busse, *Health Care Systems in Transition: Germany*, 2000.

111   Powell and Wessen, (eds.), *Health Care Systems in Transition*, 1999.

112   Federal Health Ministry, *Health Care in Germany*, website - 2001; Reimbursement and pricing of medical devices in Germany, 2000.

113   Federal Health Ministry, *Health Care in Germany*, website - 2001; and Busse, *Health Care Systems in Transition: Germany*, 2000.